The Gluten-Free Bible

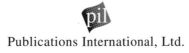

Publications International, Ltd.

Recipe development on pages 28, 30, 34, 36, 108, 110, 126, 132, 142, 204, 216, 218 and 220 by Marilyn Pocius.

Recipe development on pages 19, 90, 92, 98, 116, 122, 124, 128 and 140 by Rebecca Reilly.

Photography on pages 26, 29, 35, 37, 39, 43, 49, 51, 61, 63, 88, 91, 93, 109, 11, 113, 117, 120, 123, 125, 127, 129, 133, 135, 137, 139, 143, 150, 165, 182, 185, 189, 191, 195, 197, 205, 207, 211, 214, 217, 219, 221 and 227 by PIL Photo Studio.
Photographer: Tate Hunt
Photographer's Assistants: Stephen Pettinger, Annemarie Zelasko
Food Stylists: Kathy Joy, Carol Smoler
Assistant Food Stylists: Brittany Culver, Sheila Grannan

Ingredient photography by Christopher Hiltz.

Pictured on the front cover *(top to bottom):* Strawberry Shortcake *(page 90)* and Fiesta Beef Enchiladas *(page 198).*
Pictured on the back cover *(counterclockwise from top):* Chocolate Cupcakes with Creamy White Frosting *(page 98),* Chocolate and Pistachio Macarons *(pages 216 and 218)* and Cinnamon Raisin Bread *(page 128).*

Contributing Writer: Marilyn Pocius

Cover and title page illustration and photography on pages 4, 5, 8, 9, 14, 15, 20 and 21 by Shutterstock.
Photography on page 6 by Fotofolio.
Photography on pages 7 and 23 by Jupiterimages Unlimited.
Photography on pages 7 and 11 by iStockphoto.

ISBN-13: 978-1-60553-723-8
ISBN-10: 1-60553-723-3

Library of Congress Control Number: 2010925559

Manufactured in China.

8 7 6 5 4 3 2 1

Microwave Cooking: Microwave ovens vary in wattage. Use the cooking times as guidelines and check for doneness before adding more time.

Note: This publication is only intended to provide general information. The information is specifically not intended to be a substitute for medical diagnosis or treatment by your physician or other health care professional. You should always consult your own physician or other health care professionals about any medical questions, diagnosis, or treatment. (Products vary among manufacturers. Please check labels carefully to confirm that the products you use are free of gluten.) **Not all recipes in this book are appropriate for all people with celiac disease, gluten intolerance, food allergies or sensitivities.**

The information obtained by you from this book should not be relied upon for any personal, nutritional, or medical decision. You should consult an appropriate professional for specific advice tailored to your specific situation. PIL makes no representations or warranties, express or implied, with respect to your use of this information.

In no event shall PIL, its affiliates or advertisers be liable for any direct, indirect, punitive, incidental, special, or consequential damages, or any damages whatsoever including, without limitation, damages for personal injury, death, damage to property, or loss of profits, arising out of or in any way connected with the use of any of the above-referenced information or otherwise arising out of the use of this book.

Publications International, Ltd.

Introduction

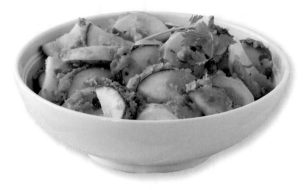

Recipes

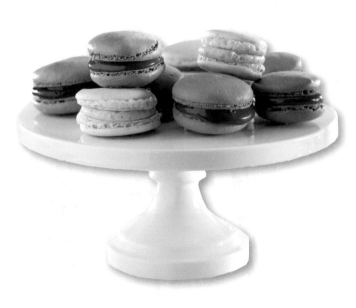

Understanding Gluten

What Is Gluten Anyway?

It's not just wheat. Gluten is a protein that is found naturally in wheat, rye and barley. Gluten gives structure to the baked goods we know and love. Without it, or something to replace it, bread and cake would be sad little puddles or piles of crumbs. When yeast, baking powder or other leavening agents produce bubbles in a dough or a batter, that air is trapped by the stretchy gluten network and the baked product rises and becomes light.

Legend has it that gluten was discovered by 7th century Buddhist monks who were trying to find something to replace the texture and savor of meat in their vegetarian diets. They found that when they submerged dough made with wheat flour in water, the starch washed away. What was left behind was a gummy mass with an almost meatlike texture—gluten. Today gluten is still used to make seitan, mock duck and other meat replacement products.

Some Techie Talk

To be technically accurate, wheat gluten is composed of two proteins—gliadin and glutenin. The proteins that make up gluten in rye and barley have different scientific names but behave much the same way since they are closely related to wheat. You will sometimes hear "corn gluten" or "rice gluten" mentioned. These proteins are very different and present no problem to those with sensitivity to wheat gluten.

Celiac Disease, Gluten Intolerance and Wheat Allergies

There are many reasons people choose to avoid gluten and many forms of gluten intolerance. Celiac disease is one of the most serious. In the 1% of Americans diagnosed with this autoimmune disorder, exposure to even small amounts of gluten can cause intestinal damage and result in symptoms from fatigue to anemia and bone disease. It is estimated that millions more may have undiagnosed celiac disease—as many as 1 out of every 133 Americans.

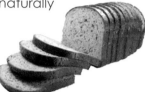

Whether you have celiac disease or another form of gluten intolerance it's good to understand the distinction. Celiac disease is a very specific condition in which exposure to gluten causes the villi, or small hairlike projections from the small intestine, to become atrophied. The purpose of these villi and the spaces between them is to let the body absorb nutrients and keep out toxins. With celiac disease, the immune system sees fragments of gluten as toxins and reacts by attacking not only the gluten but the villi themselves. An autoimmune disease, such as celiac, occurs when the body attacks itself, mistaking normal, healthy tissue for dangerous bacteria or viruses. There are more than 80 autoimmune disorders, including rheumatoid arthritis and lupus. Most, like celiac disease, are difficult to diagnose since they present a bewildering array of symptoms.

The symptoms of celiac disease and gluten sensitivity are the same. This is not surprising since they both stem from an inability to digest gluten properly. What is surprising is that there are so many different seemingly unrelated symptoms. Most people first think of gastrointestinal distress as a sign of gluten intolerance, but symptoms may also include fatigue, weight loss, weight gain, migraine headaches, anemia and sinusitis! (See the sidebar for a longer, though still not complete, list of the more than 250 possible symptoms.) Because digestion is central to providing our bodies with energy, gluten intolerance and celiac disease are multi symptomatic. Any individual may have one or many of the possible symptoms. In fact, you can have celiac disease with no symptoms at all.

It's Complicated

Just as there are many symptoms, there are many degrees of gluten sensitivity and each person's tolerance can change over time. It is possible to develop celiac disease any time in your life for any number of reasons, including enduring a stressful period. Remember, celiac is defined as damage to the intestinal villi. You could have a genetic predisposition for the disease, which only shows up under certain circumstances. Nobody knows whether what starts out as gluten intolerance can lead to celiac disease. There are also some people who are allergic to wheat itself. A classic wheat allergy is quite different from gluten intolerance. It is likely to cause the same sorts of immediate symptoms as other food allergies—itchiness, difficulty breathing and in some cases, anaphylactic shock.

On the Other Hand, It's Simple.

Millions of Americans are going gluten-free for dozens of reasons. Some have been told that they must by their doctors. Others just feel better when they stop eating gluten. Some parents feel that a gluten-free diet improves the behavior patterns of their children,

A Not-So-Short List of Possible Symptoms

Gastrointestinal:

abdominal pain or bloating
acid reflux (GERD)
constipation
diarrhea
esophagitis
heartburn
irritable bowel syndrome
nausea
vomiting
weight loss or weight gain

Other:

acne
anemia
anxiety
canker sores
depression, irritability
dermatitis
eczema
fatigue
hair loss
inability to concentrate
infertility
irregular menstrual cycles
lactose intolerance
muscle cramps
nosebleeds
respiratory problems
sinusitis
vitamin deficiencies
  (B12, K, folate)

including those with ADHD and autism. And there are those who just think it's trendy. Truth is, if giving up gluten didn't improve so many lives, people wouldn't be willing to make the effort. There is one caveat: if you want to try gluten-free living but haven't been tested for celiac disease, you need to be tested BEFORE you start the diet. Otherwise test results will be meaningless.

Testing, Testing, One, Two, Three

Why aren't we all tested for gluten intolerance automatically? And why does it often take years to come up with a diagnosis? Part of the problem has been lack of awareness, especially in the U.S. Some European countries require children to be tested by age five and most diagnose celiac disease in a matter of months. The average time between seeing a doctor and diagnosis in the U.S. can be more than ten years, but things are improving. More doctors and medical centers are devoting some of their treatment and research to celiac disease. Unfortunately, there is no one easy, sure-fire test to detect it.

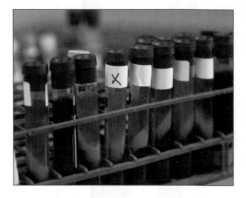

Blood samples can determine if you produce antibodies to gluten (provided you are still consuming it for several months before blood is drawn). There are five commonly used measures. None of them, unfortunately, will prove without the shadow of a doubt that you have celiac disease. If any of them is positive, your doctor may recommend a biopsy by way of endoscopy. If this determines your villi are damaged, then there is no doubt that you have celiac disease and must go on a gluten-free diet for life.

It is possible to be genetically predisposed to celiac disease, too. If you have the disease in your family, the chances are greater that you will be affected. There is also a test for genetic markers for celiac disease. If you are lacking those genes, you won't get celiac. However, not everyone who has those genes will get sick.

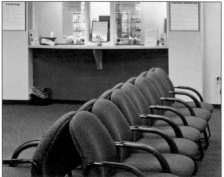

Your best resource is a doctor or clinic with experience in gluten intolerance and celiac disease. Just remember—if you stop eating gluten before the tests, they will be useless. On the other hand, if you feel better when you don't eat gluten, maybe test results aren't that important.

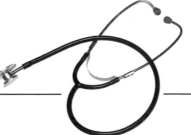

How Can Wheat Suddenly Be Bad for Us?

How could the staff of life turn into a health hazard? Is going gluten-free just the latest diet fad? It's wise to remember that the vast majorily of the population can eat all the gluten they want and never have a problem. Those with gluten intolerance simply cannot and it does seem that their number is increasing.

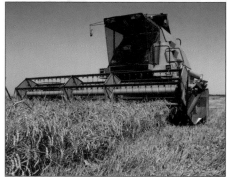

Although no one knows for sure, one factor may be that our diet today is dominated by grain, something our long-ago ancestors lived without. Wheat can feed large populations a large number of calories on relatively little land with modern agricultural methods. Of course, it also tastes good!

If you think that you don't eat much gluten because you don't eat a lot of bread, think again. Gluten in different forms is in all sorts of processed foods. It is used as a meat substitute, a filler and to improve the texture of everything from bubble gum to ketchup. So chances are you are consuming a lot more gluten than your great grandparents. Could that be why a recent study done by the Mayo Clinic found that gluten intolerance is four times more common today than it was in the 1950s?

Living Without

Eliminating gluten from your life is not easy, nor is it a short-term proposition. There is no pill for gluten intolerance and no treatment other than changing your diet for good. On the other hand, feeling healthy and energetic for the first time in years can be a huge reward for the effort. At first glance, the list of what you must give up can seem daunting—pasta, bread, crackers, bagels, pretzels, pizza, donuts, even chicken nuggets! The good news is that there are many more foods on the gluten-free list than on the forbidden one. There are also more products, from cereals to baking mixes to pastas, which are now being formulated in gluten-free versions. These days you'll find them not just in health food stores and on websites, but also on the shelves of major supermarkets.

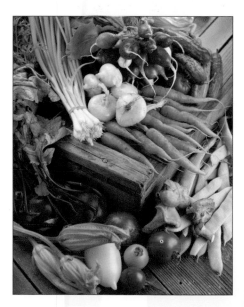

Eating gluten-free can mean eating a healthier diet—more fruits and vegetables, less processed food. You may be forced out of your old routine into doing more cooking at home and trying out new ingredients. With a bit of help from the recipes in this book, you just might find your new life is full of delicious surprises.

THE GLUTEN GUESSING GAME

It's hard enough to eliminate the obvious gluten in your life. What makes the journey tougher is that gluten hides in many places you'd never expect. Try playing our Gluten Guessing Game to test your knowledge.

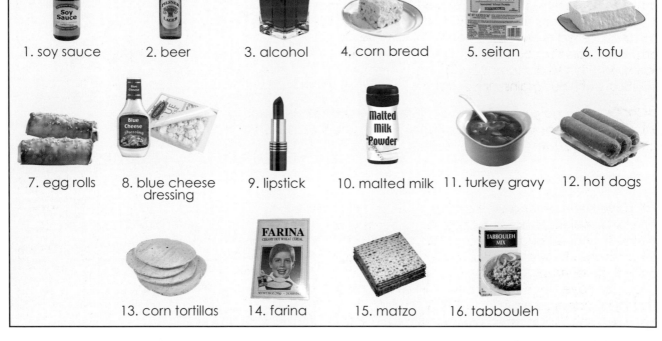

1. soy sauce
2. beer
3. alcohol
4. corn bread
5. seitan
6. tofu
7. egg rolls
8. blue cheese dressing
9. lipstick
10. malted milk
11. turkey gravy
12. hot dogs
13. corn tortillas
14. farina
15. matzo
16. tabbouleh

Answers: Numbers 2, 4, 5, 7, 10, 11, 14, 15 and 16 contain gluten. Numbers 3, 6 and 13 do NOT contain gluten. Numbers 1, 8, 9 and 12 are "maybes."

Number 1: Soy sauce is usually made with wheat; however there are some brands that are gluten-free. Tamari, which is a kind of Japanese soy sauce, is sometimes gluten-free, but read the label carefully.

Number 8: Blue cheese dressing is generally gluten-free. Blue cheese was questionable for many years since it is made with a mold that can be derived from bread. Recent studies have shown that it is safe. Even if the starter contains wheat, the gluten remaining in the finished product is practically undetectable. Some prepared salad dressings can contain other kinds of gluten, though, so check labels.

Number 9: Lipstick and other cosmetics may contain gluten. Since lipstick is most likely to be ingested, it's wise to check the label.

Number 12: Most, but NOT all, hot dogs and other sausages are gluten-free. Once again, it's important to check the labels.

Don't Despair if You Didn't Ace the Test

You'll quickly get the hang of spotting the most obvious offenders—anything with "wheat" in its name. The most confusion arises from ingredients that are derived from gluten-containing grains. These culprits most often show up in processed foods. You never have to worry about fresh fruits, veggies, meats or poultry.

If giving up wheat seems too difficult, remember that many of the world's great cuisines barely use wheat at all. Rice and soy are the basis for Asian cooking. Native Americans relied on what they called the "three sisters," corn, beans and squash. In fact, wheat is a relatively recent addition to our foodways. There are many delicious, nutritious grains and starches that can replace it.

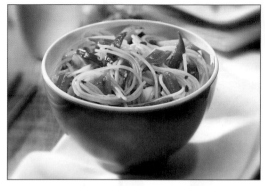
Curried Noodles
(page 70)

The best way to go gluten-free is to make the switch to a better overall diet. Start by checking out the red light/green light chart of foods on the next page.

The Never-Ending Oat Controversy

Oats have been on and off the gluten-free list for years. The main problem is that most oats are processed in facilities that also handle wheat products and are contaminated for that reason. There are brands of certified gluten-free oats available (at a premium price) that have been farmed, processed and packed in a dedicated facility. These are safe for most everyone. However, there seems to be a small subset of celiac patients who have a problem with a protein present in oats. Research is still underway.

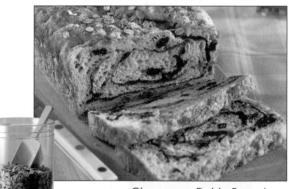
Cinnamon Raisin Bread
(page 128)

No More Crying in Your Beer

Beer lovers can rejoice! Since beer is traditionally made with barley, it used to be off limits to the gluten intolerant. These days more and more small craft brewers as well as major companies are tapping into the huge market for gluten-free products. They're brewing beer made from sorghum, millet, rice and other grains. There are already at least half a dozen breweries in the U.S. alone so you should be able to fill a frosty mug to your liking.

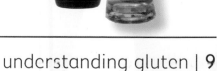

THE SHORT LIST
Sensitivities differ from person to person and ingredients differ from brand to brand. Always check the label's fine print. This is an abbreviated list of some of the most commonly used items.

RED LIGHTS: (contain gluten)

barley	couscous	imitation seafood	pretzels
beer	durum	kamut	rye
bran	einkorn	malt vinegar	seitan
brewer's yeast	emmer	malt, malt flavoring, malt extract	semolina
bulgur	graham	matzo	spelt
cereal	gravies and sauces	orzo	tabbouleh
commercial baked goods	groats (barley or wheat)	pizza	wheat
	hydrolyzed wheat protein		

Yellow Lights: (may contain gluten)

artificial color*	emulsifiers	marinades	pasta sauce
baking powder	flavorings	modified food starch*	salad dressings
barbecue sauce	frozen vegetables with sauce/seasonings	mustard	soba noodles
caramel color*	hydrolyzed plant protein (HPP)	nondairy creamer	soy sauce
dextrins*		oats (see page 9)	vegetable broth

*These items are gluten-free if made in the U.S. or Canada

Green Lights: (no gluten)

almond flour	corn, cornmeal	meat and poultry	sorghum flour
baking soda	corn grits	millet	soy, soy flour
beans	corn tortillas	mono and diglycerides	sweet rice flour (glutinous rice flour)
buckwheat	dairy	nuts	tapioca
carob	distilled alcohol	oils and fats	tofu
carrageenan	eggs	polenta	vegetables (fresh, canned or frozen without sauce/ seasonings)
cellophane noodles (bean thread noodles)	fruit, fresh, frozen or dried	potatoes	
cheese	guar gum	quinoa	vinegar (except malt)
chickpea flour (garbanzo flour, besan flour)	lentils	rice, rice flour	xanthan gum
	maltodextrin	rice noodles	
	masa harina	seafood	

ADVANCED LABEL READING

Spotting the gluten in foods is considerably easier now than ever before. Since 2004, the FDA's Food Allergy Labeling Law has required that any product containing wheat or derived from it must say so on the label. This means that many ingredients that used to be questionable, such as modified food starch and maltodextrin, must now show wheat as part of their name if they were made from it (for example, "wheat maltodextrin"). This law also applies to all eight of the most common allergens—eggs, fish, milk, peanuts, tree nuts, shellfish, soybeans and wheat. The only catch is that some sources of gluten, namely barley and rye, are NOT common allergens and don't have to be labeled. Also, you need to be aware that this ONLY applies to foods produced in the U.S. and Canada. Imports are a different matter.

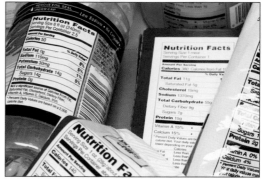

Becoming a Label Detective

Going gluten-free means you may have to start bringing a magnifying glass on your shopping trips. At the very least, you will learn a great deal about the many ingredients that go into all the processed food most of us take for granted. You may even decide that paying attention to the ingredients list is a lot more relevant than some of the marketing hype that appears on the front of the package.

The red flag you're searching for is the word "wheat." If anything in the product contains, or is made from wheat, by law it must be listed as such. Next, look for any ingredients you don't recognize. Chances are you'll find a few multisyllabic words that sound like they came from the chemistry lab. You'll need to check a list of safe and unsafe ingredients to figure those out. (You can even download such lists for your smart phone these days. See **www.celiac. com** for information.)

Soon enough, you'll recognize the most common ones that can be a problem (even if you never do learn how to pronounce them).

Codex Alimentarius: No, It's Not a Secret Society

The Codex standard is set by the Codex Alimentarius Commission, which is a joint effort of the UN and the World Health Organization. This group defines when a food product can be considered gluten-free for international trade. The current standard requires that the gluten content must not exceed 20 parts per million.

Once Is Not Enough

Product formulations change frequently. Don't assume just because you've used a brand or product in the past it is necessarily safe forever. Don't hesitate to contact the manufacturer if you have questions about ingredients. Most companies are eager to accommodate their gluten-free customers. Call the customer service help line or visit the website. You'll get the information and maybe even a few coupons for your trouble.

Does a Gluten-Free Label Mean 100% Gluten-Free?

The short answer is not exactly. Experts agree that food can contain a very small amount of gluten and still be tolerated by even those who are sensitive. The trouble is, not everyone agrees on exactly what that tiny amount should be.

The FDA is doing studies and soliciting consumer input on a definition for gluten-free which will eventually govern what appears on labels. For international trade, standards have been set at less than 20 parts per million so that is often the assumed threshold. Meanwhile, there is a private, not-for-profit certification program in place that tests products to see if they contain less than 10 parts per million of gluten. Those that do are allowed to display a "Certified Gluten-Free" logo. Remember, most food is naturally gluten-free. There's no need to look for GF labels on dairy products or a can of beans!

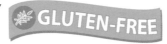

GLUTEN-FREE NUTRITION

Is Gluten-Free Healthier?

If you are suffering from celiac disease or gluten intolerance it certainly is! One of the many devastating effects can be the inability of damaged intestines to derive the nutrients your body needs. However, there are steps you should take to ensure you get proper nutrition on a gluten-free diet. Begin by talking to your doctor. Chances are, he or she can suggest a nutritionist you can consult who specializes in gluten-free eating.

The Saga of Soy Sauce

Traditional Chinese soy sauce is brewed from soybeans and wheat, so it's off limits. There are some brands that skip the brewing process and use soy concentrate and caramel coloring instead. The good news is that these GF soy sauces are cheaper, but they do lack flavor and complexity.

Tamari is a particular kind of Japanese soy sauce. Some tamari does contain wheat, however, there is a major brand that offers a certified gluten-free, wheat-free tamari. Another option is to substitute a liquid amino concentrate available at health food stores. Bottom line is always check the label!

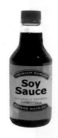

Top 10 Tips for Healthier GF Eating

1. Don't gorge on GF brownies and cookies, even when you find some that are delicious.

2. Remember that "gluten-free" on the label doesn't always mean it's healthy.

3. Don't overdo starches like rice, potatoes and corn.

4. Eat gluten-free whole grains—brown rice, whole grain cornmeal, quinoa, etc.

5. In flour mixes, look for nutritious amaranth, millet, buckwheat, montina, sorghum or teff flour.

6. Get enough fiber from whole fruits, beans, lentils and chickpeas.

7. Go global. Asian, South American, Mediterranean and Indian cuisines offer many nutritious and gluten-free dishes and ingredients.

8. Stock your kitchen and your pantry with quality ingredients and cooking equipment.

9. Get your B vitamins. In your old life, enriched white flour provided some of them. Ask your doctor if you should take a supplement.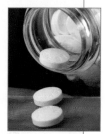

10. Protein is important and it's gluten-free! Enjoy lean meats, seafood and tofu.

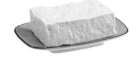

Gluten-Free Is Not Low-Calorie, Fat-Free or Low-Carb

It is most certainly not a weight-loss regimen. If you simply replace the old white bread, cakes and cookies with gluten-free versions of the same thing, you might be worse off! Most ordinary white flour is fortified to make up for the nutrients lost during processing. Some processed gluten-free flours are nutritionally empty starches. For instance, white rice flour has considerably fewer B vitamins, iron and folate than enriched white flour. It does have more refined carbohydrate, though—not a good trade-off!

On the other hand, going gluten-free can be the start of a healthier diet. You will certainly be paying more attention to the food you eat, which is a huge step in the right direction. Instead of trying to replicate your old diet, start fresh—eat more fresh fruits, vegetables, lean meat and low-fat dairy. If that sounds familiar, it is. It's the basic dietary advice given to everyone, gluten-free or not. Think of your GF lifestyle as an opportunity to try new things, not a life sentence that will deprive you of foods you used to love.

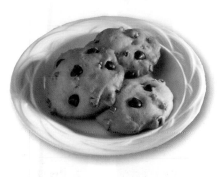

Weighing In on Gluten-Free

Some people gain weight after going gluten-free, some lose. Many newly diagnosed celiac patients are sickly and undernourished because of their disease. Once their bodies begin healing, they regain weight and strength. As gluten-free eating has become mainstream, some people try it hoping to lose weight. As with most popular diets, this is only successful if you are eating fewer calories and replacing empty ones with food that is more nutritious.

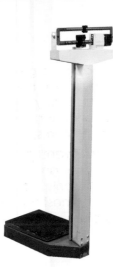

THE GLUTEN-FREE KITCHEN

How to Start Your New Life

Eating gluten-free means the days of ordering a pizza or picking up a bucket of fried chicken for dinner at the last minute are over. Don't despair! You are about to encounter a whole new world of flavors and good things to eat. GF cooking isn't difficult—it's just different. The biggest change may be that you need to cook more and use processed foods less.

For those recently diagnosed with celiac disease, setting up the kitchen to avoid cross contamination is an important first step. If you live alone, purge your place of breads, pastas, flours and other no-no's. If you are living with gluten-eating others, you'll need to stake out a GF zone of your own. The biggest culprit in cross-contamination is the common crumb. Crumbs from regular bread find their way onto work surfaces, into condiment jars and toasters. You will have to clearly mark GF items and make sure everyone understands they are hands-off. Dishes and pots and pans can be shared, because they can be washed between uses. If you will be toasting GF and regular bread, you may want to invest in a second toaster to make your life easier.

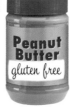

Supermarket Savvy

Before you rush off to buy a cupboard full of specialty products, remember that most basic ingredients are naturally gluten-free. You can pick up any sort of fresh produce, meat or fish without worrying. However, macaroni and cheese from a box and fish sticks are no longer on your list. This doesn't mean you can't have your favorite foods anymore. It just means you will be making some adjustments.

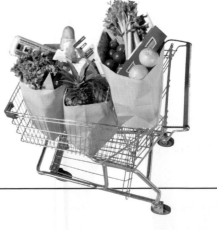

Wheat-Free Is Not Gluten-Free

When you find a product marked gluten-free you can be sure you're in safe territory. Wheat-free, however, is no guarantee. The product could contain gluten from barley, rye, oats or something derived from them. Remember, wheat is considered an allergen and must be labeled. The others are not.

Impulse shopping isn't a great option either. Most supermarkets stock huge displays with brightly colored boxes of highly processed, gluten-filled items. It may also amaze you how many aisles you can skip when you no longer wander aimlessly amidst the latest bread, cracker and snack items.

Of course, you will want to stock up on certain things so that you're prepared to eat well on your new diet. Five years ago a health food store was the only place to buy specialty flours and mixes. Fortunately, today most supermarkets offer just about everything you need. There are also many reliable online sources that are worth checking out.

THE GLUTEN-FREE PANTRY

Cooking gluten-free is easier if you keep these staples on hand.

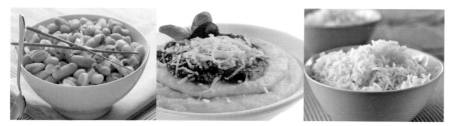

- ❑ beans and lentils
- ❑ chickpea flour
- ❑ corn grits
- ❑ corn tortillas and taco shells
- ❑ cornmeal and cornstarch
- ❑ GF cereal (corn and/or rice)
- ❑ GF flour blends (page 19)
- ❑ GF mixes for your favorite brownies, cookies or muffins
- ❑ GF pasta in various shapes

- ❑ GF soy sauce
- ❑ polenta
- ❑ quinoa
- ❑ rice (arborio rice, basmati rice)
- ❑ rice flour (brown, white and sweet rice flour)
- ❑ rice noodles
- ❑ tapioca flour
- ❑ wild rice
- ❑ xanthan gum

What Is Xanthan Gum Anyway?

It sounds mysterious, doesn't it? Xanthan gum is a chain of polysaccharides (for the nonchemists that's a chain of sugars) made by fermenting a carbohydrate (often corn sugar). Xanthan gum was approved for use as a food additive in 1968 and is used as a thickener and stabilizer in salad dressings, ice cream, low-fat dairy products and, of course, gluten-free baked goods.

In the Thick of It

From apple pie to white sauce, wheat flour is often used to thicken things. That's partly because it's cheap and readily available. There are plenty of gluten-free substitutes that offer real advantages. Tapioca flour, arrowroot and sweet rice flour (mochiko) thicken sauces and pie fillings beautifully. They also tolerate freezing and thawing better than those thickened with flour or cornstarch.

Keeping Expenses Under Control

The first time you see the price on a package of xanthan gum or gluten-free pretzels you may feel faint. Many people complain about the cost of going gluten-free, but there are ways to control spending. The biggest budget busters tend to be specialty goods, such as gluten-free cookies, cakes and snacks. It's comforting to see familiar goodies that are made just for you, and tempting to overindulge, but plenty of your old favorites are naturally gluten-free, including most potato chips, corn chips and candy.

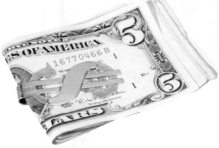

Because gluten-free is a hot topic, there are also some products that have always been gluten-free now sporting a gluten-free label and costing more. Don't pay extra for vanilla extract that's labeled gluten-free when all vanilla is!

Once you figure out which gluten-free ingredients you will need in quantity—for example flours for blends—buy in bulk. You will find many grains available in the bulk bins at the supermarket. It pays to search out online sources, as well. You can purchase millet or almond flour for a lot less per pound in a five-pound bag. If you don't have a need or the storage space for big quantities, share a shipment with gluten-free friends.

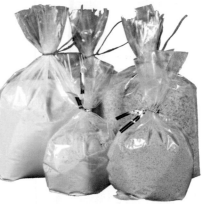

Many cultures and millions of people around the world thrive on diets with little or no gluten. In fact, ethnic markets are often great sources for well-priced gluten-free foods. Rice flour will cost less at an Asian grocer since it is in much greater demand. The same holds true for cornmeal at a Latin American market or polenta at an Italian deli. Instead of only trying to find gluten-free versions of the same old foods, use the diet as an opportunity to explore new ones.

Simple Trade-Offs

Instead of...	Try...
breakfast oatmeal	Breakfast Quinoa (page 36)
English muffins	Arepas (page 30)
chicken nuggets	Flourless Fried Chicken Tenders (page 102)
mac & cheese	Cheese Soufflé (page 204)
egg rolls	Vietnamese Summer Rolls (page 194)
Mexican carry-out	Spinach & Mushroom Enchiladas (page 202)
peanut butter cookies	Flourless Peanut Butter Cookies (page 244)

COOKING GLUTEN-FREE AND EASY

There's no need to give away your old cookbooks and recipe cards. Many recipes don't have any problematic ingredients or can easily be converted. When small quantities of flour are needed—for example, to bread chicken or fish—you can substitute any gluten-free flour for regular flour. Stock up on ready-made GF pastas and your old Italian favorites are easy as ever.

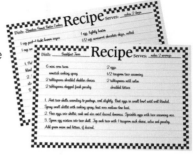

Baked goods, especially breads, are a whole lot trickier. While it is certainly possible to buy pre-made GF cookies, cakes and breads, they are expensive and can't compete with homemade treats. Fortunately, it is possible to turn out luscious gluten-free brownies, birthday cakes, pies and even bread with the recipes in this book and a bit of practice. In fact, warm GF bread from your oven is probably tastier and better for you than most supermarket wheat breads!

Flour Power

You won't be surprised to learn that the trick to making GF baked goods is finding a way to replace the power of gluten. In order to replicate the structure and texture it provides, you'll need to combine different nonwheat flours and add xanthan gum. While you can buy premade GF all-purpose flour blends as well as mixes for anything from pancakes to chocolate cake, it's helpful to know a little about the actual flours in them. It seems there are new choices available every day—hemp flour and pea flour are two of the latest. Here are descriptions of some of the more common ones.

Almond Flour has a sweet, nutty flavor that complements cookies and cakes. You can make your own almond flour by pulverizing blanched nuts in a food processor. It is very easy to end up with almond butter, though, so beware! Almond flour is low in carbohydrates and high in protein. It is a classic ingredient in Passover cooking and French macarons (pages 216–221).

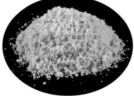

Chickpea Flour is also called garbanzo flour or besan flour. This hearty flour is high in protein, fiber and calcium. You'll find it in many Indian, Italian and Mediterranean recipes and it is an excellent addition to flour blends.

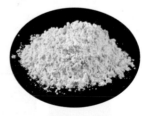

Coconut Flour is low in carbohydrates and high in fiber. It has a subtle coconut fragrance and flavor. Coconut flour absorbs a lot of liquid and can easily become dense. Recipes usually call for a small amount of coconut flour and more eggs than usual.

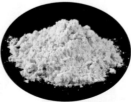

Corn Flour is the finely ground form of cornmeal. Masa harina, which is milled from hominy (corn treated with slaked lime) is a special kind of corn flour used to make tortillas and in other Mexican recipes. There is also a special corn flour used to make arepas (page 30), which is precooked and also labeled masarepa or masa al instante.

Cornmeal comes in a variety of grinds and colors, from fine to coarse, and in white, yellow and even blue! It's perfect for corn muffins, polenta and breading among other things. Cornmeal is nutritious and has a nutty, sweet flavor. Using too coarse a grind can produce gritty baked goods.

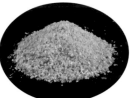

Cornstarch has probably always been in your pantry. A fine white powder, cornstarch is highly refined and used as a thickener and a bland ingredient that lightens many GF flour blends.

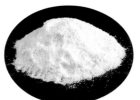

Millet Flour is made from a cereal grain that is used in African and Indian cuisine. (Whole millet is also used as bird food!) It is mild in flavor and easy to digest. Millet's mild flavor, plus a high fiber and protein content make it work well in blends for yeast breads.

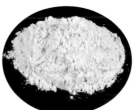

Rice Flour (white or brown) is the most commonly used gluten-free flour and a good one-to-one substitute in recipes that only call for a tablespoon or two of regular flour. Like the rice it is made from, brown rice flour is whole grain, so it is nutritionally better, but makes things heavier.

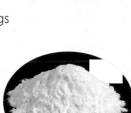

Rice Flour, Sweet can be confusing, since it's sometimes called glutinous rice flour! It does not contain gluten, but is made from short grain "sticky" rice. The Japanese term for this flour is mochiko since it is used in making mochi (rice cakes). It is an excellent thickener but has little nutritional value.

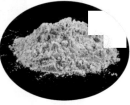

Sorghum Flour is sometimes called milo or jowar flour, and is a relatively new and very welcome addition to the gluten-free pantry. It is nutritious and high in protein so it works well in flour blends for breads. Many find the flavor similar to regular wheat flour.

Soy Flour is ground from roasted soybeans. Choose defatted soy flour. Regular is extremely perishable and prone to rancidity. Soy flour is high in protein, but it has a distinctive "beany" flavor many people don't like.

Tapioca Flour is often labeled tapioca starch. It comes from the root of the cassava (manioc) plant. You are probably more familiar with tapioca pearls used to make pudding, which come from the same root but are processed differently. Tapioca flour gives a bit of chewiness to GF baked goods and is also an excellent thickener.

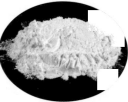

FLOUR BLENDS AND FRIENDS

Why can't there be a single one-for-one substitute for wheat flour? Unfortunately wheat flour performs many different functions and is made up of both protein (the gluten) and starches. It helps make pie crust flaky, cookies chewy and breads crusty. There is no one GF flour that can recreate all those benefits, but that's no reason to give up baking. With two basic flour blends in your refrigerator you can turn out yummy cakes, cookies and even yeast breads. Here are the blends used for many of the recipes in this book.

GLUTEN-FREE ALL-PURPOSE FLOUR BLEND

(This blend is for all baked goods not made with yeast.)

- 1 cup white rice flour
- 1 cup sorghum flour
- 1 cup tapioca flour
- 1 cup cornstarch
- 1 cup almond flour or coconut flour

Combine all ingredients in a large bowl. Whisk to make sure the flours are evenly distributed. The recipe can be doubled or tripled. Store in an airtight container in the refrigerator.

GLUTEN-FREE FLOUR BLEND FOR BREADS

(This blend is for recipes that call for yeast.)

- 1 cup brown rice flour
- 1 cup sorghum flour
- ¾ cup millet flour*
- 1 cup tapioca flour
- 1 cup cornstarch
- ⅓ cup instant mashed potato flakes (unflavored)

*If millet flour is not available, chickpea flour may be substituted.

Combine all ingredients in a large bowl. Whisk to make sure flours are evenly distributed. The recipe can be doubled or tripled. Store in an airtight container in the refrigerator.

Fiber Factoids

Most of us don't get enough fiber in our diets. Here's a list of some common GF flours and their fiber content, from high to low.

FLOUR	FIBER PER 1 CUP
Chickpea flour	20.9 grams
Almond flour	14.7 grams
Millet flour	10.3 grams
Brown rice flour	7.3 grams
White rice flour	3.8 grams
Cornstarch	1.2 grams
Tapioca	0 grams

Blending the Rules

While gluten-free flour blends may seem mysterious at first, they do follow certain logical rules. Basic all-purpose flour blends usually start with 2 parts of grain flour (rice, sorghum or millet), 2 parts of starch (cornstarch or tapioca flour) and 1 part of protein (a bean or nut flour). There are many other considerations. Flavor is one. Nutrition is also important. While a blend made of white rice flour and cornstarch might work, it wouldn't contain much in the way of fiber, protein or vitamins. You can, of course, purchase ready-made blends at the supermarket or on the Internet, but homemade is certainly cheaper and also fresher and better tasting.

Storing and Using GF Flour Blends

Most gluten-free flour blends should be stored in the refrigerator or freezer since they contain perishable whole grain or nut flours. Invest in canisters or use clearly marked resealable freezer bags. Bring flours to room temperature before using and remember to rewhisk or shake them so that they are completely combined.

Measuring GF blends is no different than measuring wheat flour, but it is even more important to be accurate. Never pack flour into a measuring cup. Don't dip the measuring cup into the flour, either, since that can compact it. Fluff the flour and spoon it into the cup. Level off the top with the back of a knife.

BAKING TIPS AND TRICKS

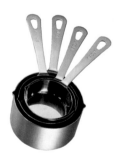

Gluten-free baking isn't harder, it's just different. The good/bad news is that you'll probably be doing more baking now that you're gluten-free. That's good because you won't be eating all the high-fructose corn syrup and other questionable ingredients in most packaged breads and cookies. The bad news is that you'll have to find the time. There is a bit of a learning curve to gluten-free baking, so don't be discouraged by a failure. Remember, you probably failed at traditional baking a few times, too! Many products that may not look as beautiful as you would like will still taste very good. You can also turn a total failure into gluten-free crumbs to be used another time.

Think Different

Many batters and doughs look drastically different from their gluten-containing counterparts. They tend to be wetter and stickier. Bread dough is more like a thick, stretchy batter. You can celebrate the fact that you'll never need to knead GF bread dough. That's a good thing, since it's so sticky you'd never be able to! You will need to learn to shape sticky dough by using damp hands or a well-oiled spoon or spatula. Parchment paper can be a real help for lining pans and transporting soft doughs.

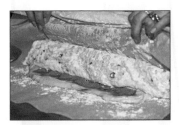

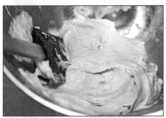

You will be using xanthan gum to provide elasticity and hold doughs together. It's important to measure it very carefully. Too much and your baked goods will shrink after baking. You may find a dense, gummy layer of dough near the bottom of the pan.

Smarty Pans

Pans are a critical part of the recipe. Black or dark metal pans can be a problem because they absorb heat more quickly. The recipes in this book were tested in pans and on baking sheets with light, shiny surfaces. If you must use dark pans, try lining them with foil, watch carefully and lower oven temperatures or cooking times if necessary. Disposable aluminum pans work surprisingly well for many recipes.

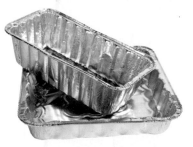

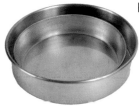

Pan size can be the difference between a perfect cake or loaf and a flop—literally! The same batter intended for a 9×5-inch loaf pan, can puff up over the top of an 8×4-inch pan and then collapse. Measure pan size across the top from inside edge to inside edge.

Temperamental Temperatures

Oven temperatures are also important. If you don't have an oven thermometer, you may want to get one. Home ovens are frequently off by as much as 50 degrees. While you're at it, pick up an inexpensive instant-read thermometer, too. It's a big help in knowing when bread is done (190° to 200°F). Gluten-free goods tend to brown more quickly. They can look done on the outside when they're still gooey in the center so be ready to cover things with a sheet of foil to prevent burning.

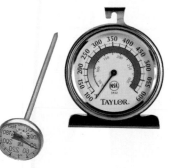

Trouble-Shooting

Problem: The cake looked gorgeous when it came out of the oven, but it fell in the center and got mushy.

Solution: Gluten-free baked goods need to be removed from pans quickly or the residual steam can cause them to collapse. Remove them from the pan to a wire rack 5 minutes after they come out of the oven.

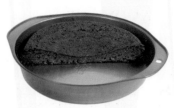

Cake left in a hot pan too long can collapse.

Problem: The muffins collapsed over the top of the pan.

Solution: There may have been too much liquid in the batter. Gluten-free flours absorb less liquid than wheat flour.

Problem: The bread was dry and hard the next morning.

Solution: GF breads stale very quickly. Always keep them well wrapped once they're cool and store in the refrigerator or freezer.

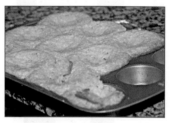

Too much liquid can make muffins collapse.

Problem: The bread was burned outside but raw in the middle.

Solution: Try lowering the oven temperature by 25 degrees. Don't bake GF breads in black, glass or nonstick-coated pans. If the outside is browning too fast, cover the bread with foil.

Problem: The cookies crumbled!

Solution: Did you remember the xanthan gum? Without it GF flours lack the elasticity to hold regular baked goods together

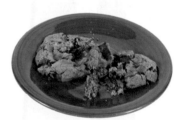

Without xanthan gum, baked goods crumble.

Problem: The bread was tough.

Solution: Beating dough for several minutes can lighten it by beating in air. Be sure to beat for the time called for in the recipe. Using a heavy duty stand mixer may help as well. You may also need to reduce the amount of flour.

Problem: The bread looked gorgeous when it came out of the oven, but then it leaned over and folded.

Solution: Don't let your GF bread rise higher than the top of the pan and don't use too small a pan.

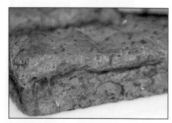

Don't let bread rise higher than the top of the pan, or it will slump.

HAPPY, HEALTHY GLUTEN-FREE KIDS

How do you explain to your child that he or she can't have a piece of Johnny's birthday cake or that those chocolate chip cookies that smell so good are off limits? It sounds impossible. Most parents would much rather make sacrifices themselves than ask their children to make them. Kids are, fortunately, considerably more resilient than we think and a gluten-free lifestyle has many positive benefits even from a pint-size perspective. Chances are this change in diet is going to be a lot harder on you than on your child.

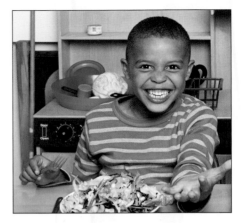

You Are Not Alone

See your doctor and make sure the right tests are done for celiac disease, gluten-intolerance and any other food sensitivities. Celiac does run in families, so if you or a close relative has the disease, it's more likely that others do as well. Seek out local support groups or search online for information and assistance in raising your gluten-free child.

Make it Positive

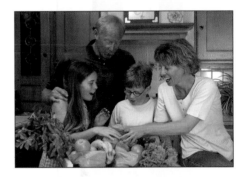

Children pick up on adult attitudes and emotions (at least until they are teenagers!). They are also quite adept at knowing when you are trying to convince them of something you don't believe. Just try to make your kid eat broccoli if you loathe it yourself! You need to appreciate the benefits of living gluten-free first. The major plus is better health now and for the future.

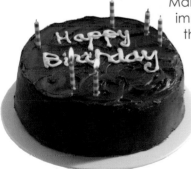

Many symptoms will improve almost immediately. Help your child understand that the reason his tummyaches went away is that he is now gluten-free. Instead of focusing on what is forbidden, emphasize the delicious gluten-free good things on the menu. Show them some of the photos of the yummy treats you'll be making from Chapter 3, "Safe Kid Stuff." They may even volunteer to help you bake.

Eight Tips to Ease the Way

1. Give Them Control. The more your child understands the GF diet and the reasons for it, the better. Sooner or later he will have to make decisions when you're not around.

2. Spread the Word. Make baby-sitters, friends' parents, relatives and school officials aware that your child is on the GF diet and that it is extremely important he sticks to it.

3. Explain How to Explain. It can be something simple, like "I'm allergic to gluten." The more a child feels comfortable talking about dietary restrictions, the safer he is.

4. Find Alternatives. You will not be able to replace brownies with broccoli. Instead bake GF brownies (page 94) or offer another gluten-free treat.

5. Party Plan. If your son or daughter is invited to a birthday party

or sleepover, send along a gluten-free replacement for whatever is being served. Explain the situation to the parent in charge and let them know what you're sending.

6. School Daze. Ask the teacher to keep a stash of gluten-free goodies on hand so when there's a celebration involving food, he won't feel left out.

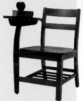

7. Use Mistakes. We all make them. If your child accidentally (or on purpose) eats gluten, don't berate him. If eating it made him feel lousy, though, point it out.

8. Don't Make it a Big Deal. It is a big deal for you, but a kid's world is filled with friends, pets, bikes, superheroes and recess. They are probably not obsessing about food like you are, and that's good.

DAIRY-FREE AND GLUTEN-FREE: THE GFCF DIET

Many families are choosing a gluten-free casein-free (GFCF) diet for children with symptoms of ADD/ADHD or autism. While there is no scientific evidence that eliminating gluten and casein helps these conditions, there are many anecdotal accounts of improvements in symptoms. Why would this be so? One theory is that some children are not able to completely digest the protein in milk (casein) and wheat (gluten) and that these leftover proteins form peptides in the blood that act like opiates in the body, influencing behavior. Research in the U.S. and Europe has found peptides in the urine of a significant number of children with autism.

Studies are currently underway to see if the GFCF diet really can be proven effective. Always consult your doctor before changing your child's diet. Tests can determine sensitivities to gluten and casein and whether there are peptides present. You should also get professional dietary advice to ensure your child will be getting the nutrition he or she needs.

What Is Casein?

Casein is the primary protein in milk. (Lactose is milk sugar. It is possible to be lactose intolerant but able to handle casein, though often when one is problematic they both are.) What complicates a GFCF diet is the fact that casein is used as a binding agent in many processed foods and goes by many different chemical names.

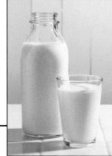

Cooking Minus the Moo

Clearly milk, cheese and butter are off the ingredient list, but did you know that most margarine contains dairy in the form of whey or casein? So do many soy cheeses. Fortunately, U.S. food manufacturers are now required to list the simple word "milk" as part of the ingredient list or in boldface type at the end of the list, even if the actual ingredient goes by an obscure chemical name. The recent popularity of the vegan diet is a boon for dairy-free shoppers, too. Since vegans consume no animal products,

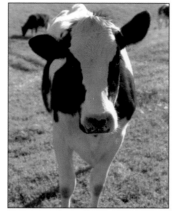

you can assume products labeled vegan are dairy-free. The kosher designation "pareve" is another handy indicator that the product contains no milk.

Nondairy is NOT Always Dairy-Free

Many products labeled nondairy contain whey, casein or other milk-derived ingredients. According to the FDA, nondairy products can contain 0.5% or less of milk products by weight. Nondairy creamers and nondairy whipped toppings usually contain dairy in some form.

Dairy Doubles

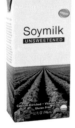

The good news is that there are more and better dairy replacement products available all the time. In addition to soymilk, you can purchase almond milk, rice milk, oat milk and even hemp milk. For most recipes, including those in this book, dairy-free milk may be substituted one-for-one for cow's milk. You may want to choose one kind of milk for drinking and another for cooking. Vanilla soymilk is delicious on its own but would be quite odd in mashed potatoes!

To replace butter in most baking recipes, choose a stick form of dairy-free margarine. Nondairy spreads sold in tubs will not always work well in baking recipes because of the softer consistency.

Cheese is one of the toughest things to replace. Some nondairy cheeses taste nothing like the real thing and many of them melt poorly or not at all, but there are more and better choices all the time. For bland cheeses, like ricotta or cottage cheese, crumbled tofu is often a good stand in.

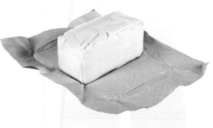

Most of the recipes in Chapter 3, "Safe Kid Stuff," are dairy-free as well as gluten-free. A special dairy-free icon marks every dairy-free recipe in the book, as well. With a bit of planning and The Gluten-Free Bible, GFCF meals can be easy, nutritious and delicious.

dairy-free

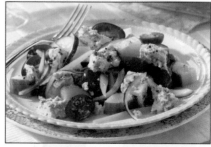

Greek Salad with Dairy-Free "Feta" (page 82)

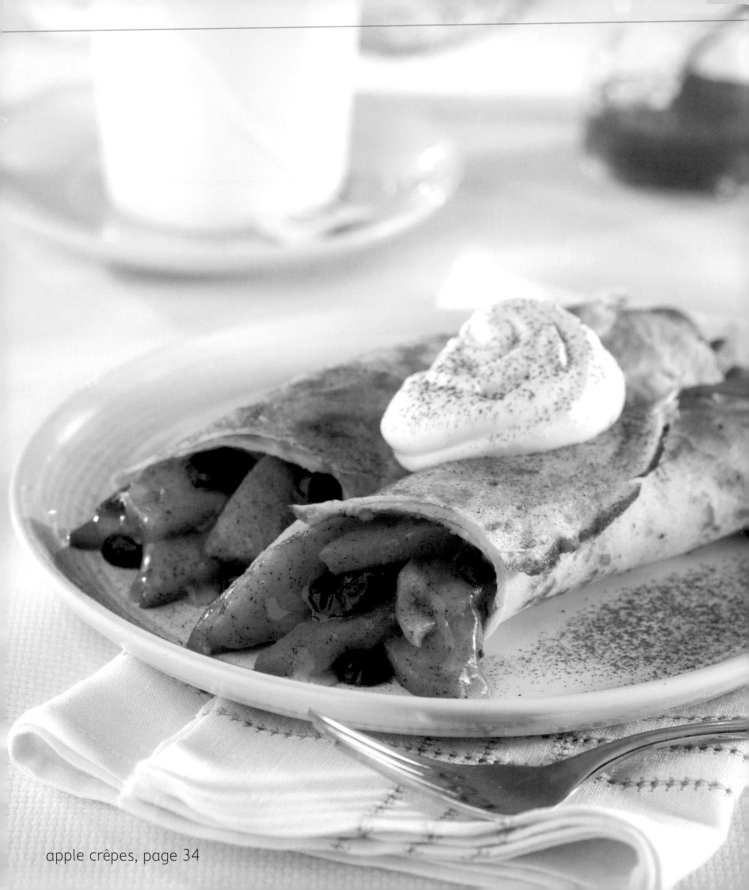

apple crêpes, page 34

smart starts

Going gluten-free is the dawn of a healthier life. Start the day right with delicious Apple Crêpes or a hearty bowl of Breakfast Quinoa with the sweet scent of cinnamon. Bet you won't miss that boring box of cereal at all.

gluten-free waffles

  2 eggs
½ cup plain yogurt
½ cup milk
  1 cup Gluten-Free All-Purpose Flour Blend (page 19)
  1 tablespoon sugar
  1 teaspoon baking powder
  1 teaspoon baking soda
½ teaspoon salt
  2 tablespoons butter, melted
    Butter and syrup

1. Preheat waffle iron according to manufacturer's directions.

2. Beat eggs in large bowl until light and fluffy. Whisk in yogurt and milk.

3. Combine flour blend, sugar, baking powder, baking soda and salt in medium bowl.

4. Gradually whisk yogurt mixture into flour mixture to make smooth batter. Whisk in melted butter.

5. Add batter to waffle iron by ½ cupfuls for 6-inch waffles (adjust amount depending on waffle iron). Bake until crisp and browned. Serve with butter and syrup. Refrigerate or freeze leftover waffles; reheat in toaster oven until crisp.   *Makes 5 (6-inch) waffles*

dairy-free variation

Replace regular yogurt with plain or vanilla soy yogurt. Replace milk with soymilk, almond milk or other dairy-free milk. Replace butter with dairy-free margarine.

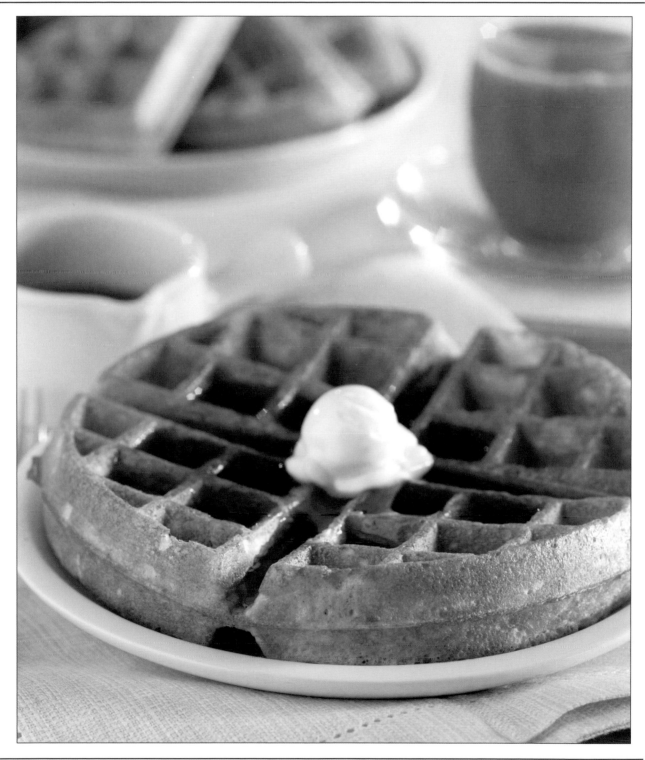

arepas (latin american corn cakes)

1½ **cups instant corn flour for arepas (see sidebar)**
½ **teaspoon salt**
1½ **to 2 cups hot water**
⅓ **cup shredded Mexican cheese blend**
1 **tablespoon butter, melted**
   Fillings: scrambled or fried eggs, cheese and salsa

1. Preheat oven to 350°F. Mix flour and salt in medium bowl. Stir in 1½ cups hot water. Dough should be smooth and moist but not sticky. Add more water by tablespoonfuls if needed. Add cheese and butter. Knead until dough is consistency of smooth mashed potatoes.

2. Preheat heavy skillet or griddle over medium heat. Grease lightly with butter or oil. Break off a piece of dough about the size of an egg; roll dough into a ball. (If dough cracks or seems too dry, return to bowl and add additional water by tablespoonfuls.) Flatten and pat into 3- to 4-inch disc about ½-inch thick. Immediately place in hot skillet.

3. Cook arepas 3 to 5 minutes per side until browned in spots. Transfer to baking sheet. Bake 15 minutes or until arepas sound hollow when tapped.

4. To make breakfast sandwiches, split arepas by piercing edges with fork as you would English muffins. Fill with eggs, cheese and salsa as desired.   *Makes 6 to 8 arepas*

note: Arepas are best served warm; day-old arepas are best toasted. Arepas may also be frozen for future use.

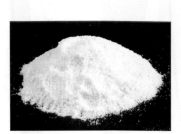

gluten-free info

The corn flour used in this recipe is also called masarepa, masa al instante and harina precodica. It is NOT the same as masa harina or regular cornmeal. Purchase arepa flour at Latin American markets or on the Internet.

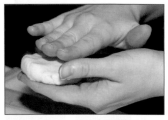

Pat the dough into a disc.

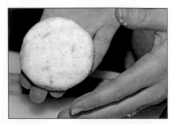

Discs should be 3 to 4 inches in diameter and ½ inch thick.

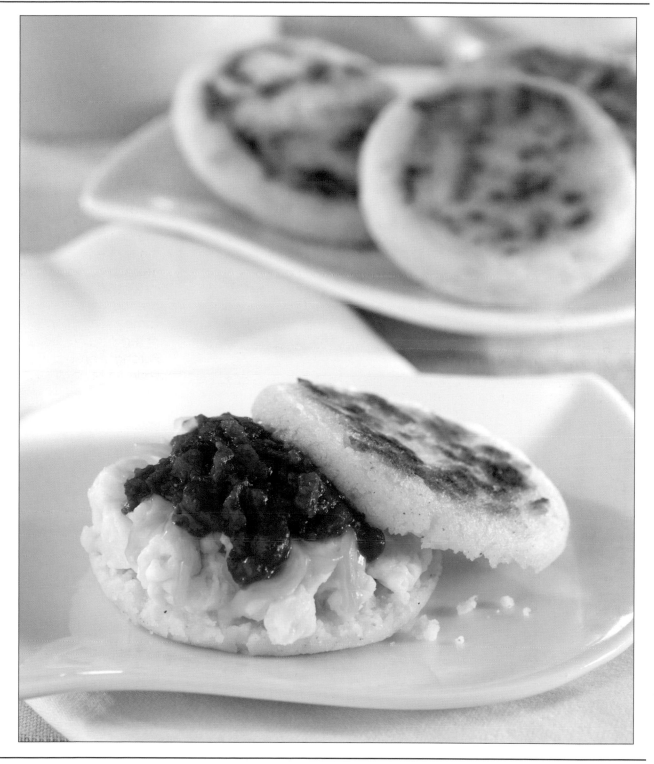

breakfast pizza

2 cups refrigerated or frozen shredded hash brown potatoes, thawed

½ cup finely chopped onion

¼ cup tomato paste

2 tablespoons water

½ teaspoon dried oregano

2 eggs, lightly beaten

½ cup (2 ounces) shredded mozzarella cheese

2 tablespoons bacon bits

1. Combine potatoes and onion in medium bowl.

2. Lightly spray medium nonstick skillet with cooking spray. Add potato mixture; flatten with spatula. Cook 7 to 9 minutes per side or until both sides are lightly browned.

3. Mix tomato paste and water in small bowl; spread evenly over potatoes in skillet. Sprinkle oregano over tomato mixture.

4. Pour eggs over potato mixture. Cover and cook 4 minutes. Sprinkle mozzarella and bacon bits over egg. Cover and cook 1 minute.

5. Slide pizza from skillet onto serving plate. Cut into wedges.

Makes 2 servings

dairy-free variation

Omit cheese; instead top with cooked vegetables or a dairy-free cheese alternative.

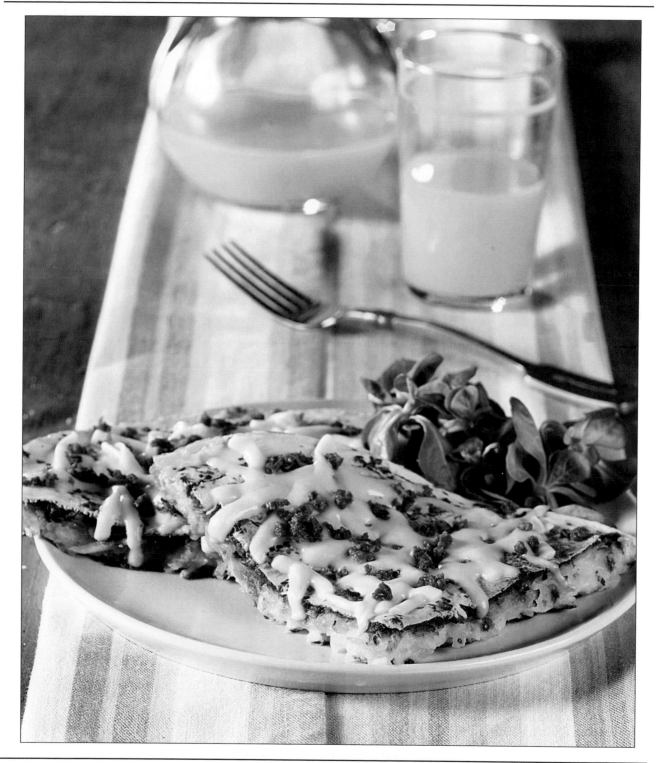

apple crêpes

[pictured on page 26]

1 cup rice flour
¼ teaspoon salt
¼ teaspoon nutmeg
1 cup half-and-half
3 tablespoons butter, melted, divided
½ teaspoon vanilla
3 eggs
Apple Filling (see sidebar)

1. Combine rice flour, salt and nutmeg in medium bowl. Gradually whisk in half-and-half until smooth.

2. Add 2 tablespoons butter and vanilla. Whisk in eggs, one at a time, until batter is smooth with consistency of heavy cream.

3. Prepare Apple Filling; keep warm.

4. Heat 8- or 9-inch nonstick skillet over medium heat. Brush lightly with some of remaining butter. Pour about ¼ cup batter into center of pan. Immediately swirl pan to coat with batter. Cook about 1 minute or until crêpe is dull on top and edges are dry. Turn and cook 30 seconds. Remove to plate; repeat with remaining batter.

5. Fill crêpes with Apple Filling. Freeze leftover crêpes between sheets of waxed paper in large resealable freezer food storage bag.   *Makes about 14 crêpes*

apple filling

Slice 5 firm apples into wedges and place in large bowl. Sprinkle with 1 tablespoon sugar and 1 teaspoon ground cinnamon. Add ¼ cup dried cranberries; toss to combine. Melt 2 tablespoons butter in large nonstick skillet over medium heat. Add apple mixture; cook and stir 5 minutes or until apples soften.

ham & potato pancakes

 dairy-free

¾ **pound Yukon gold potatoes, peeled, grated and squeezed dry (about 2 cups)**

¼ **cup finely chopped green onions**

2 **eggs, beaten**

1 **cup (4 to 5 ounces) finely chopped cooked ham**

¼ **cup rice flour**

¼ **teaspoon salt**

¼ **teaspoon black pepper**

2 **to 3 tablespoons vegetable oil**

Chili sauce or fruit chutney (optional)

1. Combine potatoes, green onions and eggs in large bowl; mix well. Add ham, rice flour, salt and pepper; mix well.

2. Heat 2 tablespoons oil in large heavy skillet over medium-high heat. Drop batter into skillet by heaping tablespoonfuls and press with spatula to flatten. Cook 2 to 3 minutes per side. Remove to paper towels to drain. Add remaining 1 tablespoon oil, if necessary, to cook remaining batter. Serve pancakes with chili sauce.

Makes 16 pancakes

gluten-free info

Rice flour can often be substituted for regular all-purpose flour in recipes like this one where a small amount of flour is called for to bind ingredients together. Use either brown or white rice flour. Brown rice flour, like the brown rice it is made from, has a slightly better nutritional profile.

breakfast quinoa

dairy-free

½ **cup quinoa**

1 **cup water**

1 **tablespoon packed brown sugar**

2 **teaspoons maple syrup**

½ **teaspoon ground cinnamon**

¼ **cup golden raisins (optional)**

Raspberries and bananas

Soymilk, almond milk or other dairy-free milk

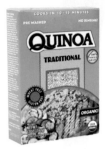

1. Place quinoa in fine-mesh strainer; rinse well under cold running water. Transfer to small saucepan. Stir in water, brown sugar, maple syrup and cinnamon. Bring to a boil. Reduce heat; simmer, covered, 10 to 15 minutes until quinoa is tender and water is absorbed. Add raisins, if desired, for last 5 minutes of cooking time.

2. Top quinoa with raspberries and bananas. Serve with soymilk.

Makes 2 servings

gluten-free info

Quinoa is an excellent gluten-free grain to know. It is relatively new to most Americans, but it has been cultivated and appreciated for 6,000 years in South America. Unlike wheat or rice, quinoa is a complete protein and is also a good source of fiber.

Tiny grains of quinoa expand to four times their size when cooked and become light and translucent.

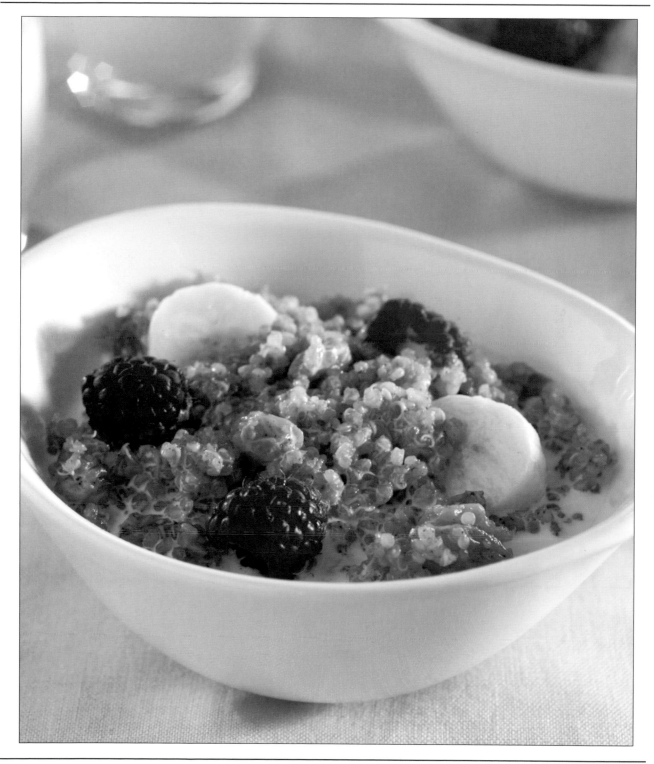

mushroom & onion egg bake

 1 tablespoon vegetable oil

 4 ounces sliced mushrooms

 4 green onions, chopped

 1 cup cottage cheese

 6 eggs

 1 cup sour cream

 2 tablespoons Gluten-Free All-Purpose Flour Blend (page 19)

 ¼ teaspoon salt

 ⅛ teaspoon black pepper

 Dash hot pepper sauce

1. Preheat oven to 350°F. Grease shallow 1-quart baking dish.

2. Heat oil in medium skillet over medium heat. Add mushrooms and onions; cook and stir 5 minutes or until tender.

3. Place cottage cheese in food processor; pulse until almost smooth. Add eggs, sour cream, flour blend, salt, black pepper and hot pepper sauce; pulse until combined. Pour into prepared baking dish. Stir in mushrooms and onions. Bake about 40 minutes or until knife inserted near center comes out clean. *Makes 6 servings*

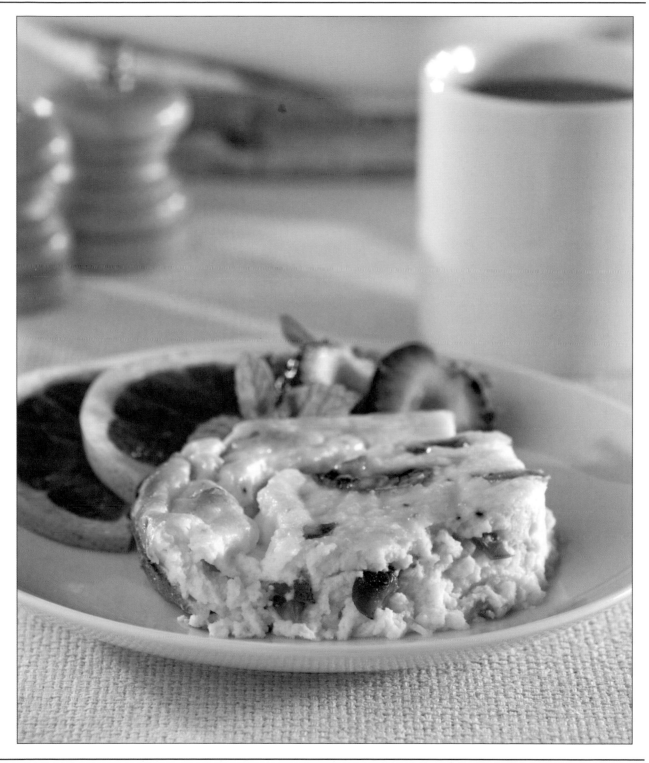

goat cheese & tomato omelet

3 egg whites

2 eggs

1 tablespoon water

⅛ teaspoon salt

⅛ teaspoon black pepper

Nonstick cooking spray

⅓ cup crumbled goat cheese

1 medium plum tomato, diced

2 tablespoons chopped fresh basil or parsley

1. Whisk together egg whites, eggs, water, salt and pepper in medium bowl.

2. Spray medium nonstick skillet with cooking spray; heat over medium heat. Add egg mixture; cook 2 minutes or until eggs begin to set on bottom. Lift edges of omelet to allow uncooked eggs to flow underneath. Cook 3 minutes or until center is almost set.

3. Sprinkle cheese, tomato and basil in center of omelet. Fold half of omelet over filling. Cook 1 to 2 minutes or until cheese begins to melt and center is set. Cut omelet in half; transfer to serving plates.

Makes 2 servings

recipe notes

Goat cheese, also called chèvre from the French, comes in many shapes and sizes. Fresh goat cheese is most often seen in a cylindrical shape, often coated with herbs or black pepper, although there are also round, square and even pyramid-shaped cheeses. The texture can range from creamy to fairly firm and the flavor from mild to sharp and a bit gamey. Try different styles until you find the ones you like best.

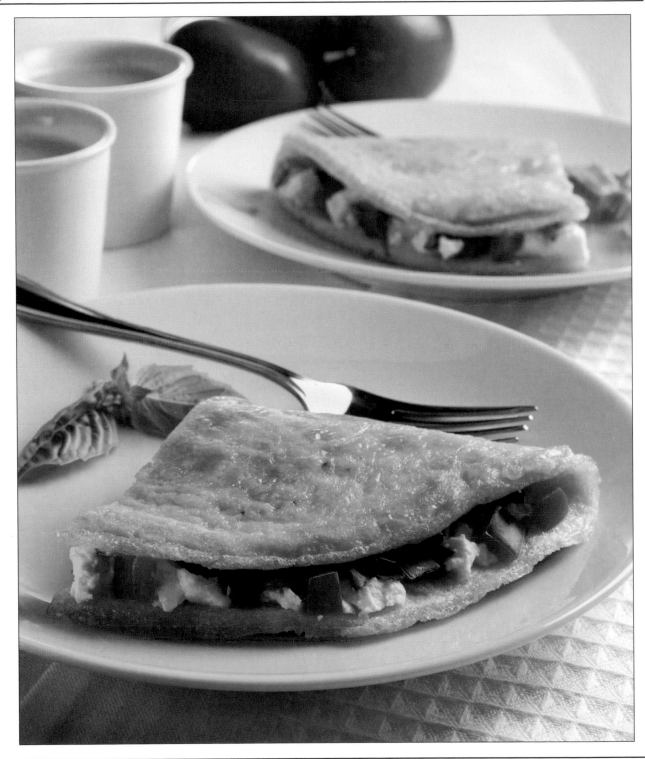

apple & raisin oven pancake

1 large baking apple, cored and thinly sliced

⅓ cup raisins

2 tablespoons packed brown sugar

½ teaspoon ground cinnamon

4 eggs

⅔ cup milk

⅔ cup Gluten-Free All-Purpose Flour Blend (page 19)

2 tablespoons butter, melted

Powdered sugar (optional)

1. Preheat oven to 350°F. Spray 9-inch pie plate with nonstick cooking spray.

2. Combine apple, raisins, brown sugar and cinnamon in medium bowl. Transfer to prepared pie plate. Bake, uncovered, 10 to 15 minutes or until apple begins to soften. Remove from oven. *Increase oven temperature to 450°F.*

3. Whisk eggs, milk, flour blend and butter in medium bowl until blended. Pour batter over apple mixture. Bake 15 minutes or until pancake is golden brown. Sprinkle with powdered sugar, if desired.

Makes 6 servings

dairy-free variation

Replace milk with soymilk, almond milk or other dairy-free milk. Replace butter with dairy-free margarine.

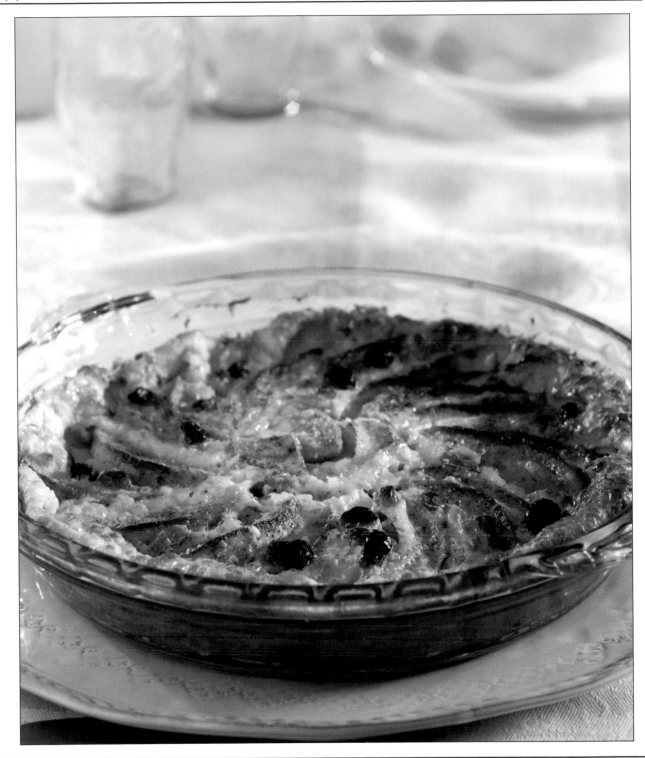

crustless ham & asparagus quiche

2 cups sliced asparagus (½-inch pieces)
1 red bell pepper, finely chopped
1 cup milk
2 tablespoons rice flour
3 eggs
1 cup chopped ham
2 tablespoons chopped fresh tarragon or basil
½ teaspoon salt
¼ teaspoon black pepper
½ cup (2 ounces) finely shredded Swiss cheese

1. Preheat oven to 350°F. Combine asparagus, bell pepper and 1 tablespoon water in microwavable bowl. Cover with waxed paper; microwave on HIGH 2 minutes or until vegetables are crisp-tender. Drain.

2. Whisk milk and rice flour in large bowl. Whisk in eggs until well blended. Stir in vegetables, ham, tarragon, salt and black pepper. Pour into 9-inch pie plate.

3. Bake 35 minutes. Sprinkle cheese over quiche; bake 5 minutes or until center is set and cheese is melted. Let stand 5 minutes before serving. *Makes 6 servings*

dairy-free variation

Replace milk with plain soymilk, almond milk or other dairy-free milk. Omit Swiss cheese or replace with dairy-free cheese alternative.

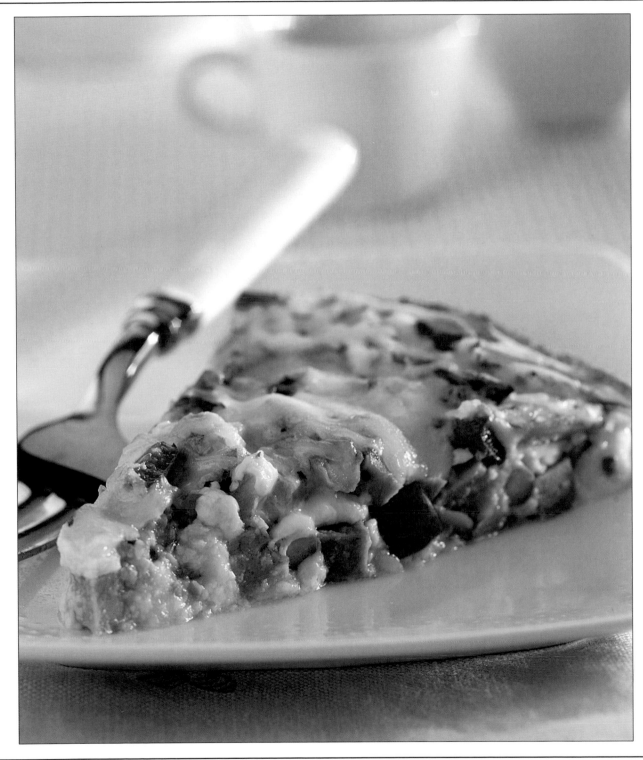

summer fruit brunch cake

 dairy-free

¾ cup Gluten-Free All-Purpose Flour Blend (page 19)

½ cup cornmeal

1 teaspoon xanthan gum

½ teaspoon baking powder

¼ teaspoon baking soda

½ cup (1 stick) dairy-free margarine, softened

⅔ cup granulated sugar

2 eggs

½ cup vanilla soy yogurt, plus additional for topping

1 cup fresh peach slices *or* 1 can (about 15 ounces) sliced peaches in juice, drained

Sliced strawberries

1. Preheat oven to 325°F. Spray 9-inch pie plate with nonstick cooking spray. Combine flour blend, cornmeal, xanthan gum, baking powder and baking soda in medium bowl.

2. Beat margarine and sugar in large bowl with electric mixer at medium speed until fluffy. Add eggs and ½ cup yogurt; beat until well combined. Beat in flour mixture until combined. Stir in peaches.

3. Pour batter into prepared pie plate. Bake 35 minutes or until toothpick inserted into center comes out clean. Serve with strawberries and drizzle with yogurt. *Makes 6 servings*

allergy info

It's a lot easier these days to enjoy the taste and health benefits of yogurt without the dairy. Soy and rice yogurt are readily available and come in a variety of flavors. Most are cultured like regular yogurt. The latest yogurt variety to hit the shelves is coconut milk yogurt. It's always wise to check the ingredients list before purchasing, especially if you have multiple sensitivities.

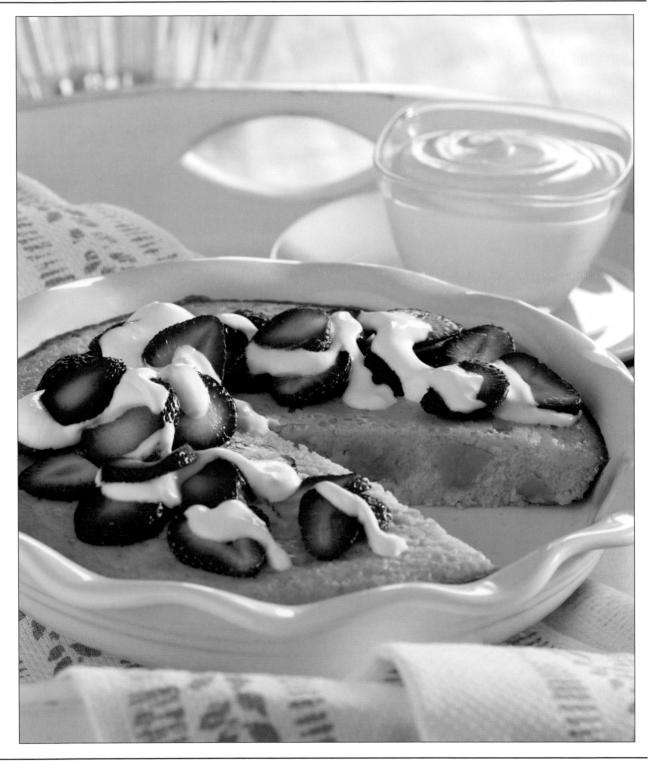

potato-zucchini pancakes with warm corn salsa

dairy-free

how-to

To shred zucchini, use the large holes on a box grater or the shredding disc of a food processor. It's best to start with zucchini that are no more than 2 inches in diameter, since bigger vegetables can be seedy or watery. Scrub them well and cut off the ends, but don't peel! The dark green peel adds color as well as nutrition. After shredding, drain the zucchini well in a colander, pressing down to remove excess moisture.

> Warm Corn Salsa (recipe follows)
> 2 cups frozen hash brown potatoes, thawed
> 1½ cups shredded zucchini, drained (see sidebar)
> 2 eggs
> ¼ cup Gluten-Free All-Purpose Flour Blend (page 19)
> 2 tablespoons chopped onion
> 2 tablespoons chopped green bell pepper
> ¼ teaspoon salt
> ⅛ teaspoon black pepper

1. Prepare Warm Corn Salsa; keep warm.

2. Combine potatoes, zucchini, eggs, flour blend, onion, bell pepper, salt and black pepper in medium bowl until well blended.

3. Spray large nonstick skillet with cooking spray; heat over medium-high heat. Drop potato mixture by ¼-cupfuls into skillet. Cook pancakes about 3 minutes per side or until golden brown. Serve with Warm Corn Salsa. *Makes 6 servings*

warm corn salsa

> Nonstick cooking spray
> 2 tablespoons chopped onion
> 2 tablespoons finely chopped green bell pepper
> 1 package (9 ounces) frozen corn, thawed
> 1 cup chunky salsa
> 2 teaspoons chopped fresh cilantro

Spray small nonstick skillet with cooking spray; heat over medium heat. Add onion and bell pepper. Cook and stir 3 minutes or until crisp-tender. Add corn, salsa and cilantro. Reduce heat to medium-low. Cook 5 minutes or until heated through. *Makes 3 cups*

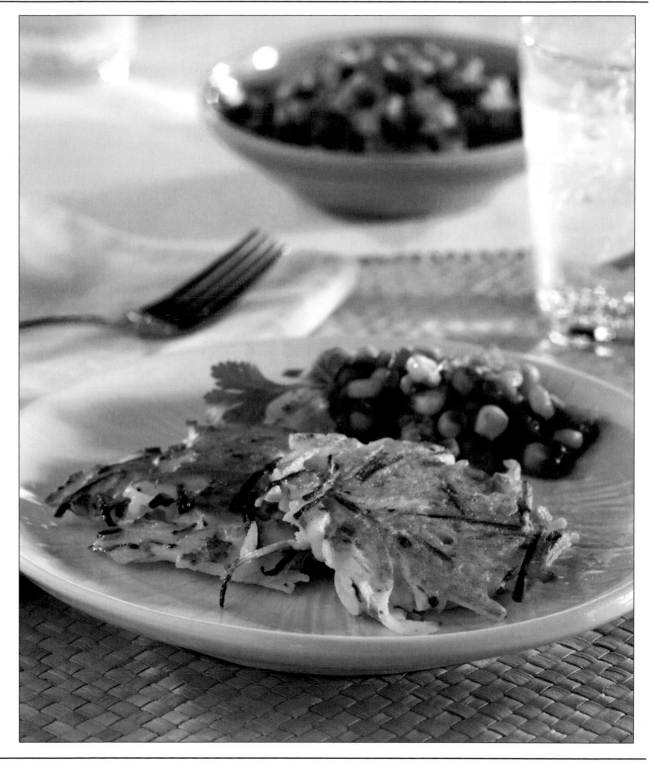

mexican omelet roll-ups with avocado sauce

Nonstick cooking spray

8 eggs

2 tablespoons milk

1½ cups (6 ounces) shredded Monterey Jack cheese

1 large tomato, seeded and chopped

¼ cup chopped fresh cilantro

8 corn tortillas

1½ cups salsa (optional)

2 medium avocados, chopped

¼ cup sour cream

2 tablespoons finely chopped onion

1 jalapeño or serrano pepper,* seeded and chopped

1 to 2 teaspoons fresh lime juice

¼ teaspoon salt

¼ teaspoon minced garlic

Jalapeño peppers can sting and irritate the skin, so wear rubber gloves when handling peppers and do not touch your eyes.

1. Preheat oven to 350°F. Spray 13×9-inch baking dish with cooking spray.

2. Whisk eggs and milk in medium bowl until blended. Spray large skillet with cooking spray; heat over medium heat. Add egg mixture; cook and stir 5 minutes or until eggs are almost set. Remove from heat. Stir in cheese, tomato and cilantro.

3. Spoon about ⅓ cup egg mixture evenly down center of each tortilla. Roll up tortillas and place seam side down in prepared dish. Pour salsa evenly over tortillas, if desired.

4. Cover tightly with foil and bake 20 minutes or until heated through.

5. Meanwhile, process avocados, sour cream, onion, jalapeño, lime juice, salt and garlic in food processor or blender until smooth. Serve roll-ups with avocado sauce. *Makes 8 servings*

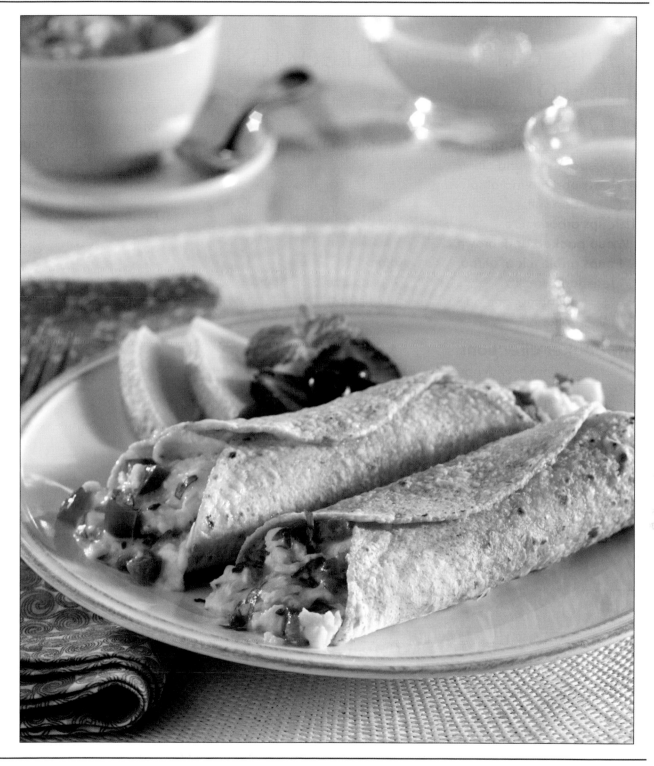

apple-cinnamon breakfast risotto

¼ cup (½ stick) butter

4 medium Granny Smith apples, diced (about 1½ pounds)

1½ teaspoons ground cinnamon

¼ teaspoon ground allspice

¼ teaspoon salt

1½ cups arborio rice

½ cup packed dark brown sugar

4 cups apple juice, at room temperature

1 teaspoon vanilla

Sliced almonds and dried cherries (optional)

Milk (optional)

slow cooker directions

1. Coat slow cooker with nonstick cooking spray. Melt butter in large skillet over medium-high heat. Add apples, cinnamon, allspice and salt. Cook and stir 3 to 5 minutes or until apples begin to release juices. Transfer to slow cooker.

2. Add rice and stir to coat. Sprinkle brown sugar evenly over top. Add apple juice and vanilla. Cover; cook on HIGH 1½ to 2 hours or until all liquid is absorbed. Top with almonds and dried cherries and drizzle with milk, if desired. *Makes 6 servings*

gluten-free info

It's good to get to know different kinds of rice to add variety to your gluten-free cooking. Arborio rice, a short grain Italian variety, is preferred for risotto. Arborio is a high starch grain. The release of some of this starch into the cooking liquid contributes to risotto's creamy texture.

dairy-free variation

Replace butter with dairy-free margarine.

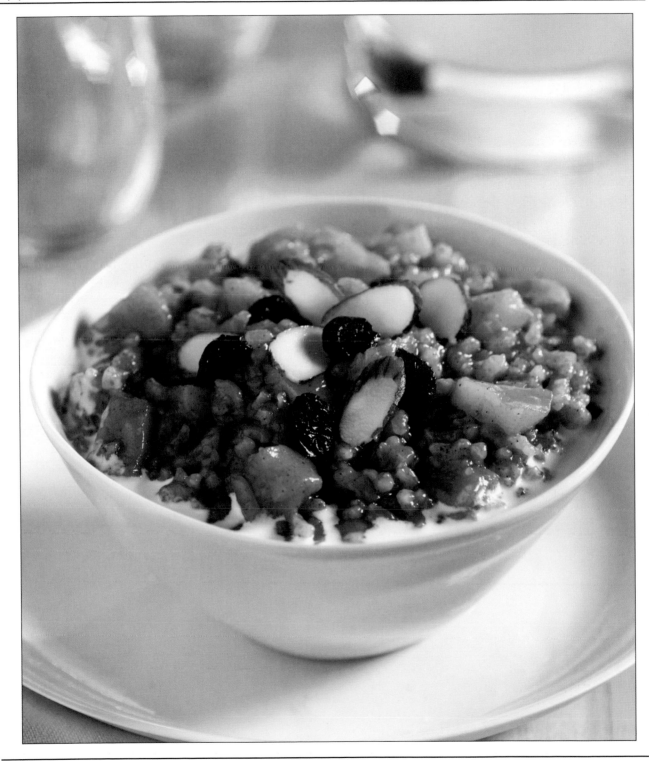

wild rice & pepper frittata

1 tablespoon olive oil
1 large shallot, minced
1 clove garlic, minced
1 cup chopped shiitake mushrooms
1 large roasted red pepper, chopped
1 cup cooked wild rice
½ teaspoon salt, divided
¼ teaspoon black pepper, divided
⅛ teaspoon ground paprika
6 eggs
¼ cup shredded Asiago cheese

1. Preheat broiler. Heat oil in large nonstick ovenproof skillet. Add shallot and garlic. Cook and stir over medium heat 1 minute. Add mushrooms; cook and stir 5 minutes or until tender. Stir in red pepper, wild rice, ¼ teaspoon salt, ⅛ teaspoon black pepper and paprika. Cook and stir over high heat 1 minute or until liquid evaporates. Remove from heat.

2. Beat eggs in large bowl with remaining ¼ teaspoon salt and ⅛ teaspoon black pepper. Pour eggs into skillet; tilt to spread over rice mixture. Cook over medium heat until eggs are almost set. Sprinkle with cheese.

3. Broil 3 to 4 minutes or until cheese melts and frittata edges are browned. Let rest 2 to 3 minutes to firm up. *Makes 6 servings*

how-to

To roast a fresh red bell pepper, place it on a stovetop over an open flame or 4 inches from heat in a broiler. Turn it frequently to blacken all sides, using long-handled tongs. Place the blackened pepper in a paper or plastic bag, close the bag and set it aside for 30 minutes to loosen the skin. Peel off the blackened skin with a paring knife or rub off with your fingers.

dairy-free variation

Omit cheese or replace with a dairy-free cheese alternative.

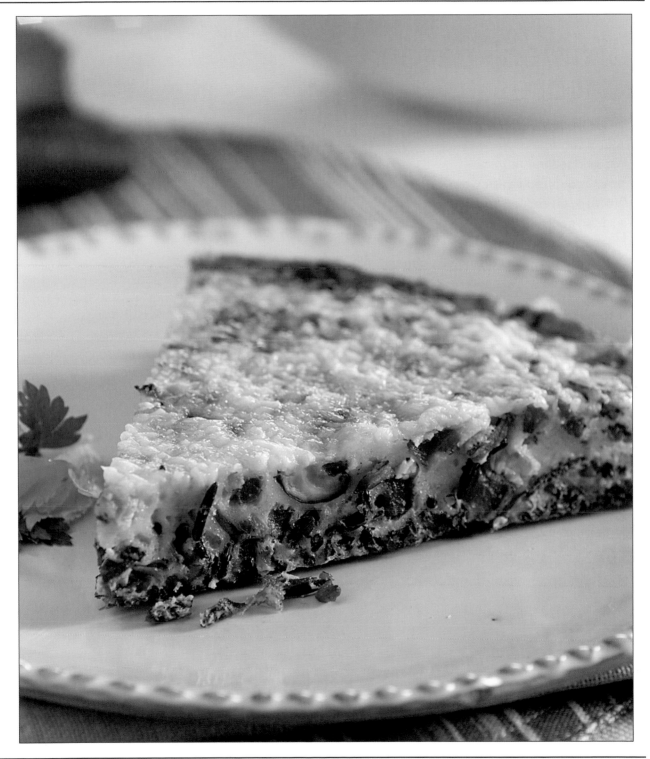

cornmeal-pecan pancakes

 dairy-free

1 cup yellow cornmeal

⅓ cup sugar

¼ cup rice flour

1 teaspoon baking powder

½ teaspoon baking soda

¼ teaspoon salt

⅛ teaspoon nutmeg

1 cup plain or vanilla soymilk, almond milk or other dairy-free milk

1 egg

1 tablespoon canola oil

½ teaspoon vanilla

¼ cup chopped pecans

Maple syrup

Nonstick cooking spray

1. Combine cornmeal, sugar, rice flour, baking powder, baking soda, salt and nutmeg in large bowl; mix well. Combine soymilk, egg, oil and vanilla in medium bowl; whisk until smooth. Add soymilk mixture to cornmeal mixture; stir until smooth batter forms. Stir in pecans.

2. Spray griddle or large nonstick skillet with cooking spray; heat over medium-high heat. Spoon 2 tablespoons batter onto hot griddle for each pancake; spread to 3-inch diameter. Cook 2 to 3 minutes or until tops of pancakes are bubbly; turn and cook 1 minute more or until bottoms are lightly browned. Serve with syrup.

Makes 8 servings

gluten-free info

Finely ground cornmeal is the best choice for this recipe. A coarser grind could cause the pancakes to have a gritty texture. Choose whole grain cornmeal instead of degerminated cornmeal. It provides better nutrition and also a deeper corn flavor. Whole grain cornmeal is available in a variety of grinds, from fine to coarse.

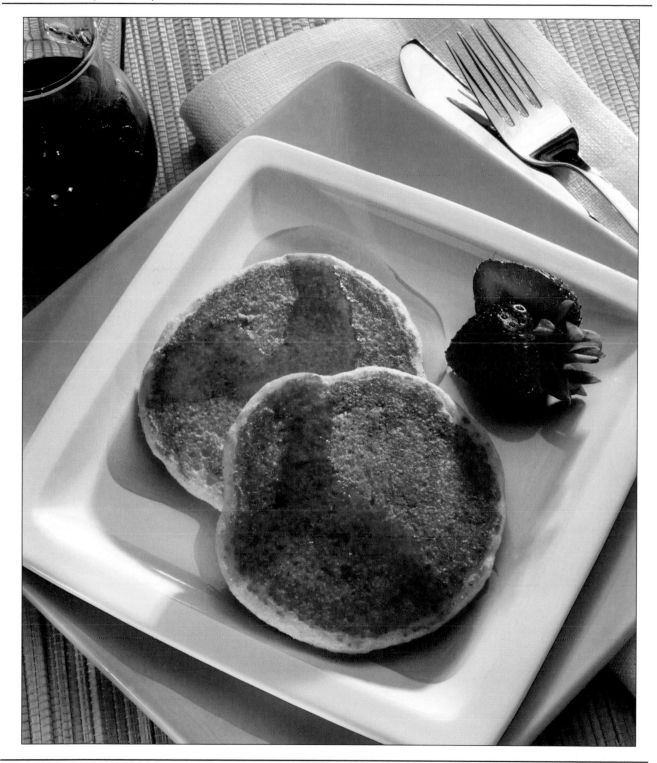

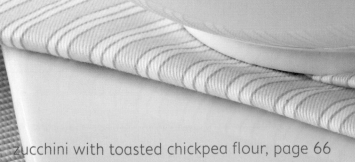

zucchini with toasted chickpea flour, page 66

small plates

When you need a starter, a snack or a light meal, you'll find it right here. The plates may be small, but the flavors aren't. Dishes like Sweet Potato Gnocchi and Savory Mexican Potato Tart will delight everyone, whether they are eating gluten-free or not.

mandarin chicken salad

dairy-free

3½ ounces thin rice noodles (rice vermicelli)

1 can (6 ounces) mandarin orange segments, chilled

⅓ cup honey

2 tablespoons rice wine vinegar

2 tablespoons gluten-free soy sauce

1 can (8 ounces) sliced water chestnuts, drained

4 cups shredded napa cabbage

1 cup shredded red cabbage

½ cup sliced radishes

4 thin slices red onion, cut in half and separated

3 boneless skinless chicken breasts (about 12 ounces), cooked and cut into strips

1. Place noodles in large bowl; cover with hot water. Soak 15 to 20 minutes or until soft. Drain and set aside.

2. Drain mandarin orange segments, reserving ⅓ cup liquid. Whisk together reserved liquid, honey, vinegar and soy sauce in small bowl. Add water chestnuts.

3. Combine Napa and red cabbages, radishes and onion in medium bowl. Divide noodles among four serving plates. Top evenly with cabbage mixture, chicken and orange segments. Remove water chestnuts from dressing and arrange on salads. Drizzle with remaining dressing.

Makes 4 servings

gluten-free info

Rice noodles are semi-translucent dried noodles that come in many sizes and have many names, including rice stick noodles, rice-flour noodles and pho noodles. Widths range from string thin (usually called rice vermicelli) to 1 inch wide. All rice noodles must be soaked to soften before using and all may be used interchangeably.

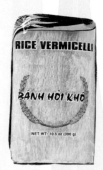

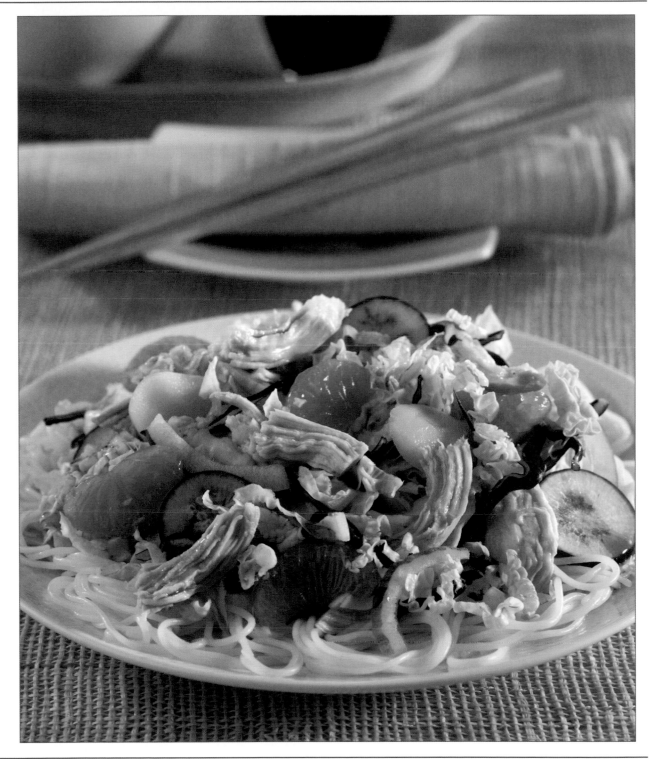

cheese blintzes

1 cup rice flour
¼ teaspoon salt
¼ teaspoon nutmeg
1 cup half-and-half
3 tablespoons butter, melted, divided
½ teaspoon vanilla
3 eggs
1 container (15 ounces) ricotta cheese
2 tablespoons powdered sugar
1 teaspoon vanilla
Preserves, applesauce or sour cream

1. Combine rice flour, salt and nutmeg in medium bowl. Gradually whisk in half-and-half until smooth.

2. Add 2 tablespoons butter and vanilla. Whisk in eggs, one at a time, until batter is smooth with the consistency of heavy cream.

3. Heat 8- or 9-inch nonstick skillet over medium heat. Brush lightly with some of remaining butter. Pour about ¼ cup batter into center of pan. Immediately swirl pan to coat with batter. Cook about 1 minute or until crêpe is dull on top and edges are dry. Turn and cook 30 seconds. Remove to plate; keep warm. Repeat with remaining batter.

4. Meanwhile, combine ricotta, powdered sugar and vanilla in medium bowl. Fill crêpes with ricotta mixture. Serve with preserves, applesauce or sour cream.   *Makes about 14 blintzes*

gluten-free info

White rice flour is a better choice for this recipe since it will produce a lighter, smoother crêpe. GF crêpes freeze well and can be used in a multitude of ways. Separate the crêpes with pieces of waxed paper, stack them and store them in a plastic freezer bag. They thaw quickly and can be filled with fruit (see Apple Crêpes, page 34), cheese, jam or even served simply sprinkled with powdered sugar.

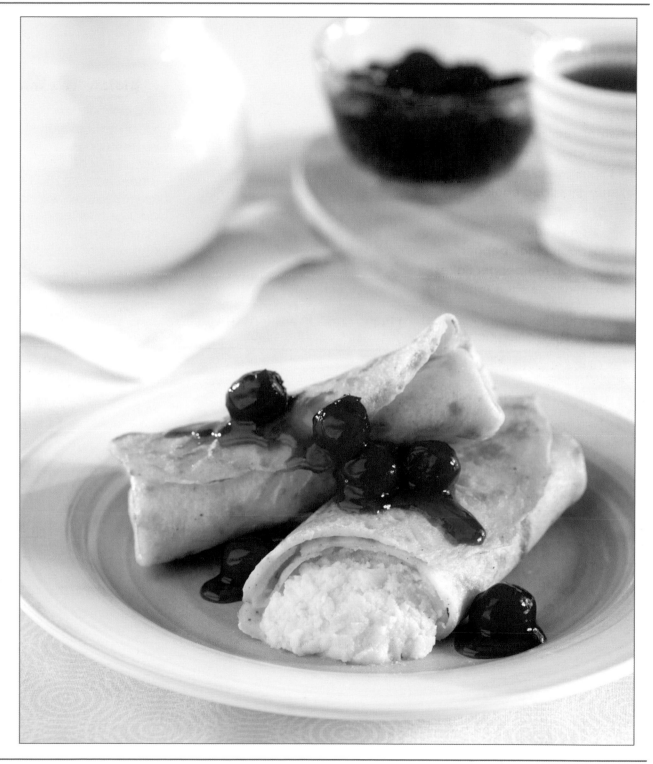

spanish tortilla

dairy-free

1 teaspoon olive oil

1 cup thinly sliced peeled potato

1 small zucchini, thinly sliced

¼ cup chopped onion

1 clove garlic, minced

1 cup shredded cooked chicken

8 eggs

½ teaspoon salt

½ teaspoon black pepper

¼ teaspoon red pepper flakes

Fresh tomato salsa (optional)

1. Heat oil in 10-inch nonstick skillet over medium-high heat. Add potato, zucchini, onion and garlic; cook and stir about 5 minutes or until potato is tender, turning frequently. Stir in chicken; cook 1 minute.

2. Meanwhile, whisk eggs, salt, black pepper and red pepper flakes in large bowl. Carefully pour egg mixture into skillet. Reduce heat to low. Cover and cook 12 to 15 minutes or until egg mixture is set in center.

3. Loosen edges of tortilla and slide onto large serving platter. Let stand 5 minutes; cut into wedges. Serve warm or at room temperature. Serve with salsa, if desired.

Makes 10 to 12 servings

gluten-free info

A Spanish tortilla (tortilla Española) has nothing in common with the Mexican tortilla, except for the fact that it's round! At its most basic, a Spanish tortilla is an open-face potato and egg omelet. In Spain these omelets are often served in tapas bars or as a light dinner.

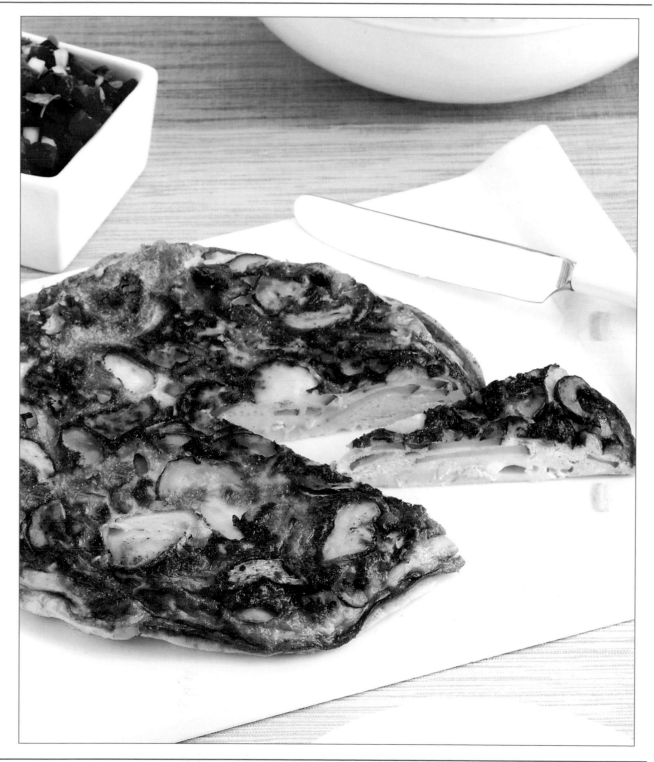

zucchini with toasted chickpea flour

[pictured on page 58]

½ **cup sifted chickpea flour (see sidebar)**
1½ **pounds zucchini or summer squash (3 or 4)**
2 **tablespoons olive oil**
1 **tablespoon butter**
3 **teaspoons minced garlic**
1 **teaspoon salt**
½ **teaspoon pepper**
½ **cup water**

1. Heat small skillet over medium-high heat; add chickpea flour. Cook and stir 3 to 4 minutes until fragrant and slightly darker in color. Remove from skillet; set aside.

2. Cut zucchini into ½-inch thick circles or half moons. Heat oil and butter in large skillet. Cook and stir garlic 1 minute or until fragrant. Add zucchini, salt and pepper; cook and stir 5 minutes or until beginning to soften.

3. Stir chickpea flour into skillet to coat zucchini. Pour in water; cook and stir 2 to 3 minutes or until moist crumbs form, scraping bottom of skillet frequently to prevent sticking and scrape up brown bits.

Makes 4 servings

gluten-free info

Using chickpea flour to add substance and nutrition to vegetable dishes is a method adapted from Indian cuisine. The flour forms delicious, nutty crumbs that become part of the dish. Try this recipe with broccoli, cauliflower or other vegetables.

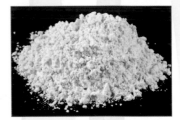

dairy-free variation

Replace butter with dairy-free margarine or additional olive oil.

falafel nuggets

dairy-free

sauce

- 2½ **cups tomato sauce**
- ⅓ **cup tomato paste**
- 2 **tablespoons lemon juice**
- 2 **teaspoons sugar**
- 1 **teaspoon onion powder**
- ½ **teaspoon salt**

falafel

- 2 **cans (15 ounces each) chickpeas, rinsed and drained**
- ½ **cup rice flour**
- ½ **cup chopped fresh parsley**
- 1 **egg**
- **Juice of 1 lemon**
- ¼ **cup minced onion**
- 2 **tablespoons minced garlic**
- 2 **teaspoons ground cumin**
- ½ **teaspoon salt**
- ½ **teaspoon ground red pepper or red pepper flakes**
- ½ **cup canola oil**

1. For sauce, combine tomato sauce, tomato paste, lemon juice, sugar, onion powder and ½ teaspoon salt in medium saucepan. Simmer over medium-low heat 20 minutes; keep warm.

2. Meanwhile, preheat oven to 400°F. Coat baking sheet with nonstick cooking spray.

3. Combine chickpeas, rice flour, parsley, egg, lemon juice, minced onion, garlic, cumin, ½ teaspoon salt and red pepper in food processor or blender; process until well blended. Shape mixture into 1-inch balls.

4. Heat oil in large nonstick skillet over medium-high heat. Fry falafel in batches until browned. Place 2 inches apart on baking sheet; bake 8 to 10 minutes. Serve with warm sauce.

Makes 12 servings

variation

Falafel can also be baked completely to reduce fat content. Spray the falafel lightly with nonstick cooking spray and bake 15 to 20 minutes, turning once.

sweet potato gnocchi dairy-free

1½ **pounds sweet potatoes (2 or 3 medium)**
¼ **cup sweet rice flour, plus additional for rolling (see sidebar)**
1 **tablespoon lemon juice**
1 **teaspoon salt**
½ **teaspoon xanthan gum**
½ **teaspoon nutmeg**
½ **teaspoon black pepper**
¼ **teaspoon sugar**
2 to 4 **tablespoons extra virgin olive oil**
1 **pound spinach, stemmed**

1. Preheat oven to 375°F. Poke sweet potatoes with fork in several places. Bake 50 to 60 minutes or until very soft. Remove and discard skins. Press potatoes through ricer or mash very well; discard stringy pieces. You should have about 2½ cups mashed sweet potato.

2. Combine sweet potato, rice flour, lemon juice, salt, xanthan gum, nutmeg, pepper and sugar in medium bowl. Mix well.

3. Heavily flour cutting board or work surface. Working in batches, scoop portions of dough onto board and roll into ½-inch-thick rope using floured hands. Cut into ¾-inch pieces. Shape each piece into oval; make ridges with tines of fork. Transfer to foil-lined baking sheet. Freeze gnocchi at least 30 minutes on baking sheet.*

4. Heat 1 tablespoon oil in large nonstick skillet. Add frozen gnocchi in batches and cook, turning once, until lightly browned and warmed through, adding additional oil as needed to prevent sticking. Keep warm.

5. Add olive oil to coat bottom of skillet. Add spinach; cook and stir 30 seconds or just until barely wilted. Serve gnocchi on bed of spinach. *Makes 4 servings*

*Gnocchi may be made ahead to this point and frozen for up to 24 hours. For longer storage, transfer frozen gnocchi to covered freezer container.

gluten-free info

Sweet rice flour is sometimes labeled glutinous rice flour (although it is gluten-free) or mochiko (the Japanese term). It is available in the Asian section of large supermarkets, at Asian grocers and on the Internet.

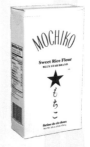

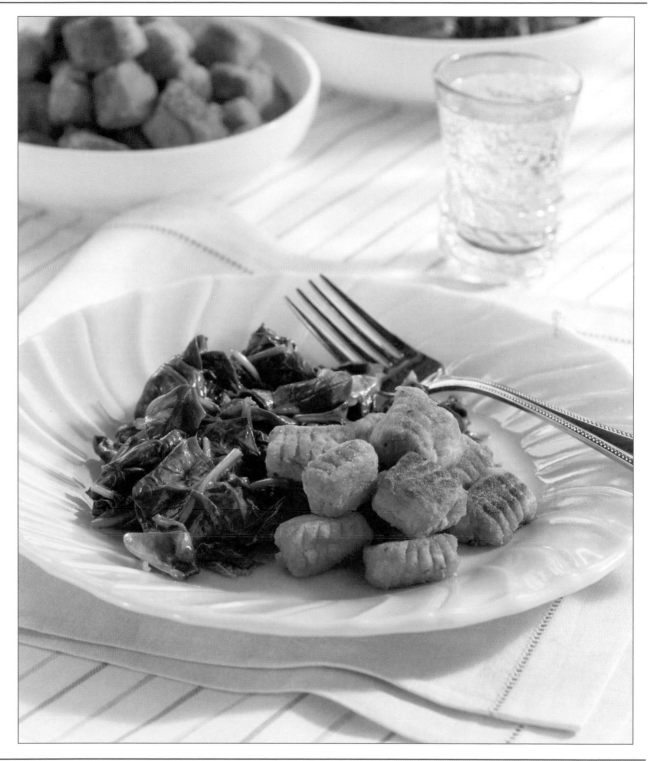

curried noodles

dairy-free

- 7 ounces thin rice noodles (rice vermicelli)
- 1 tablespoon peanut or vegetable oil
- 1 large red bell pepper, cut into short, thin strips
- 2 green onions, cut into ½-inch pieces
- 1 clove garlic, minced
- 1 teaspoon minced fresh ginger
- 2 teaspoons curry powder
- ⅛ to ¼ teaspoon red pepper flakes
- ½ cup vegetable broth
- 2 tablespoons gluten-free soy sauce

1. Place noodles in large bowl; cover with hot water. Soak 15 to 20 minutes or until soft. Drain; cut into 3-inch pieces.

2. Heat oil in wok or large skillet over medium-high heat. Add red pepper strips; stir-fry 3 minutes.

3. Add green onions, garlic and ginger; stir-fry 1 minute. Add curry powder and red pepper flakes; stir-fry 1 minute.

4. Add broth and soy sauce; cook and stir 2 minutes. Add noodles; cook and stir 3 minutes or until heated through.

Makes 6 servings

gluten-free info

Asian rice noodles are a great go-to for gluten-free diets. Most are made only of rice flour and water. Rice noodles come in various widths and are sometimes labeled rice sticks or rice vermicelli. Do check labels carefully though, since occasionally rice noodles contain wheat flour as well.

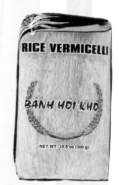

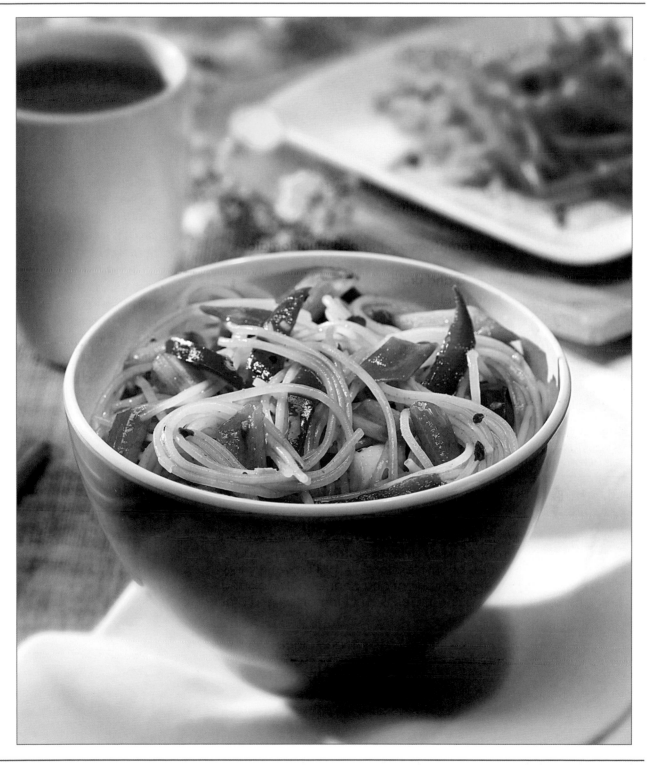

quinoa & roasted corn

 dairy-free

1 cup uncooked quinoa

½ teaspoon salt

4 ears corn *or* 2 cups frozen corn

¼ cup plus 1 tablespoon vegetable oil, divided

1 cup chopped green onions, divided

1 teaspoon coarse salt

1 cup quartered grape tomatoes or chopped plum tomatoes, drained*

1 cup black beans, rinsed and drained

¼ teaspoon grated lime peel

Juice of 1 lime (about 2 tablespoons)

¼ teaspoon sugar

¼ teaspoon cumin

¼ teaspoon black pepper

Place tomatoes in fine-mesh strainer and place over bowl 10 to 15 minutes.

1. Place quinoa in fine-mesh strainer; rinse well under cold running water. Transfer to medium saucepan; add 2 cups water and ½ teaspoon salt. Bring to a boil over high heat. Reduce heat; cover and simmer 15 to 18 minutes or until water is absorbed and quinoa is tender. Transfer quinoa to large bowl.

2. Meanwhile, remove husks and silk from corn; cut kernels off cobs. Heat ¼ cup oil in large skillet over medium-high heat. Add corn; cook 10 to 12 minutes or until tender and light brown, stirring occasionally. Stir in ⅔ cup green onions and coarse salt; cook and stir 2 minutes. Add corn to quinoa. Gently stir in tomatoes and black beans.

3. Combine lime peel, lime juice, sugar, cumin and black pepper in small bowl. Whisk in remaining 1 tablespoon oil until blended. Pour over quinoa mixture; toss lightly to coat. Sprinkle with remaining ⅓ cup green onions. Serve warm or chilled.

Makes 6 to 8 servings

how-to

Quinoa is usually rinsed before using. The seeds are naturally coated with a substance called saponin, which protects quinoa from insects while it's growing. The grain is almost always rinsed during processing to remove the bitter saponin, but it doesn't hurt to rinse quinoa again before using it. Place it in a fine-mesh strainer and swish the grains around under cold running water. If the water looks cloudy or soapy, that's the saponin.

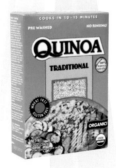

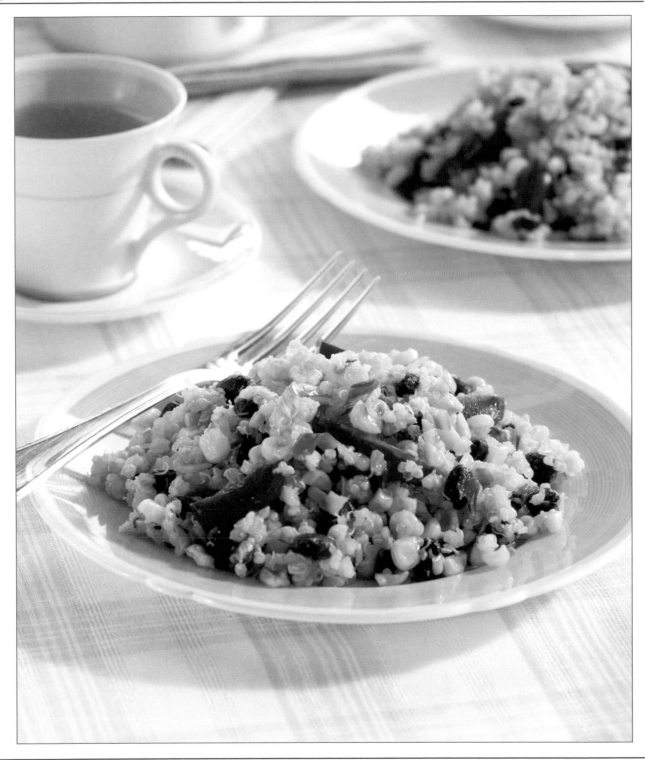

buckwheat with zucchini & mushrooms

dairy-free

1½ to 2 tablespoons olive oil
1 cup sliced mushrooms
1 medium zucchini, cut into ½-inch dice
1 medium onion, chopped
1 clove garlic, minced
¾ cup buckwheat
¼ teaspoon dried thyme
¼ teaspoon salt
⅛ teaspoon black pepper
1¼ cups vegetable broth
Lemon wedges (optional)

1. Heat oil in large nonstick skillet over medium heat. Add mushrooms, zucchini, onion and garlic. Cook and stir 7 to 10 minutes or until vegetables are tender. Stir in buckwheat, thyme, salt and pepper. Cook and stir 2 minutes.

2. Add broth; bring to a boil. Cover; reduce heat to low. Cook 10 to 13 minutes or until liquid is absorbed and buckwheat is tender. Remove from heat; let stand, covered, 5 minutes. Serve with lemon wedges, if desired.   *Makes 4 to 6 servings*

variation: For a richer flavor, add pancetta to this dish. Coarsely chop 4 slices pancetta; cook in medium skillet over medium heat about 5 minutes until crisp. Add 1 tablespoon olive oil, then add mushrooms, zucchini, onion and garlic. Proceed as directed.

gluten-free info

Buckwheat is a gluten-free grain despite the fact that "wheat" is part of its name. It is actually a fruit seed, totally unrelated to wheat, and is a cousin to garden rhubarb. Hulled buckwheat is referred to as "buckwheat groats" or "kasha" in its toasted form. Buckwheat flour is used to make soba noodles, but be cautious; most soba noodles also contain wheat flour.

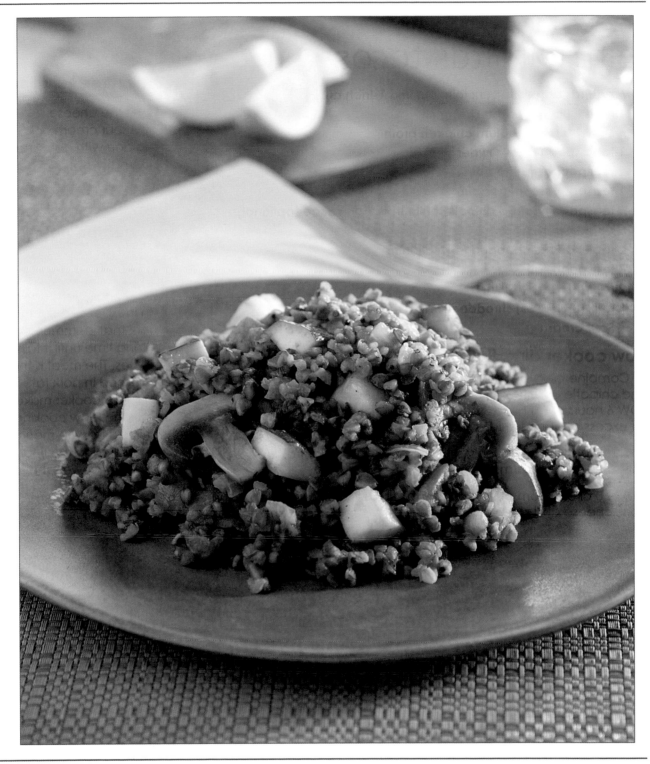

mini carnitas tacos

1½ **pounds boneless pork loin, cut into 1-inch cubes**
 1 **onion, finely chopped**
½ **cup reduced-sodium chicken broth**
 1 **tablespoon chili powder**
 2 **teaspoons ground cumin**
 1 **teaspoon dried oregano**
½ **teaspoon minced chipotle chile in adobo sauce (optional)**
½ **cup pico de gallo**
 2 **tablespoons chopped fresh cilantro**
½ **teaspoon salt**
12 **(6-inch) corn tortillas**
¾ **cup (3 ounces) shredded sharp Cheddar cheese**
   Sour cream

slow cooker directions

1. Combine pork, onion, broth, chili powder, cumin, oregano and chipotle chile, if desired, in slow cooker. Cover; cook on LOW 6 hours or on HIGH 3 hours or until pork is very tender. Pour off excess cooking liquid.

2. Shred pork with two forks; stir in pico de gallo, cilantro and salt. Cover and keep warm.

3. Cut 3 circles from each tortilla with 2-inch biscuit cutter. Top with pork, cheese and sour cream.   *Makes 36 mini tacos*

dairy-free variation

Omit the cheese and sour cream or replace with dairy-free alternatives.

recipe notes

Carnitas means "little meats" in Spanish. This dish is usually made with an inexpensive cut of pork that is simmered for a long time until it falls to pieces. The meat is then browned in pork fat. The slow cooker makes the long, slow cooking process easy to manage and skipping the final browning lowers the fat content.

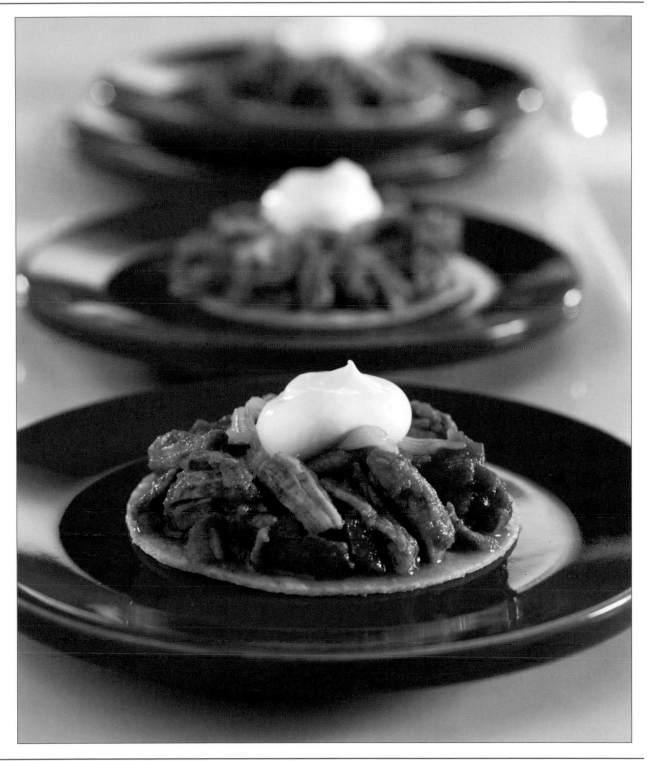

socca (niçoise chickpea pancake)

 dairy-free

1 cup **chickpea flour**

¾ **teaspoon salt**

½ **teaspoon ground pepper**

1 cup **water**

5 tablespoons **olive oil, divided**

1½ teaspoons **minced fresh basil** *or* ½ **teaspoon dried basil**

1 teaspoon **minced fresh rosemary** *or* ¼ **teaspoon dried rosemary**

¼ **teaspoon dried thyme**

1. Sift chickpea flour into medium bowl. Stir in salt and pepper. Gradually whisk in water to create a smooth batter. Stir in 2 tablespoons olive oil. Allow batter to rest at least 30 minutes.

2. Preheat oven to 450°F about 10 minutes before ready to bake socca. Place 9- or 10-inch cast iron skillet in oven to heat.

3. Add basil, rosemary and thyme to batter; whisk until smooth. Carefully remove skillet from oven using oven mitts. Add 2 tablespoons olive oil to skillet; swirl to coat evenly. Immediately pour in batter.

4. Bake 12 to 15 minutes or until edge begins to pull away and center is firm. Remove skillet; turn oven to broil.

5. Brush socca with remaining tablespoon oil and broil 2 to 4 minutes until dark brown in spots. Cut into wedges and serve warm. *Makes 6 servings*

recipe note

Socca are pancakes made of chickpea flour and are commonly served in paper cones as a savory street food in the south of France, especially around Nice. Chickpea flour can also be used to make crêpes. Increase the amount of water in the recipe by about ¼ cup to make a thinner batter and cook the crêpes in a small nonstick skillet.

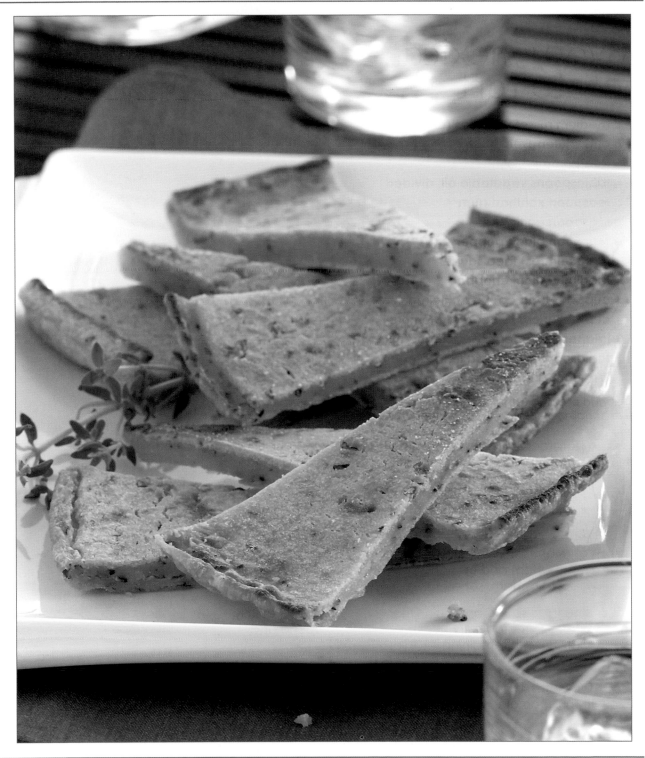

savory mexican potato tart

   3 medium russet potatoes (about 1 pound), peeled
   ½ cup Gluten-Free All-Purpose Flour Blend (page 19)
   ¼ cup cornmeal
   4 tablespoons vegetable oil, divided
   ½ teaspoon xanthan gum
   ½ teaspoon garlic salt
   ½ teaspoon black pepper
   1 jar (8 ounces) taco sauce
   1 medium onion, chopped
   1 cup shredded cooked chicken
   1 cup (4 ounces) shredded Monterey Jack cheese
   1 jalapeño pepper,* seeded and minced
   2 tablespoons chopped fresh oregano
      Prepared guacamole

Jalapeño peppers can sting and irritate the skin, so wear rubber gloves when handling peppers and do not touch your eyes.

1. Place potatoes in large saucepan; add water to cover. Bring to a boil over high heat. Reduce heat to low; cover and simmer 30 minutes or until potatoes are fork-tender. Drain. Mash potatoes in large bowl with electric mixer at low speed. Add flour blend, cornmeal, 3 tablespoons oil, xanthan gum, garlic salt and black pepper; mix until smooth.

2. Preheat oven to 350°F. Dust hands with flour blend. Press potato mixture onto bottom and up side of ungreased 10-inch tart pan with removable bottom; set aside.

3. Combine taco sauce and onion in small bowl; spread evenly over potato mixture. Top with chicken, cheese, jalapeño and oregano. Drizzle with remaining 1 tablespoon oil.

4. Bake 30 minutes or until potato mixture is heated through. Cool in pan 10 minutes. Loosen edge of tart with knife. Remove rim. Serve with guacamole.   *Makes 8 servings*

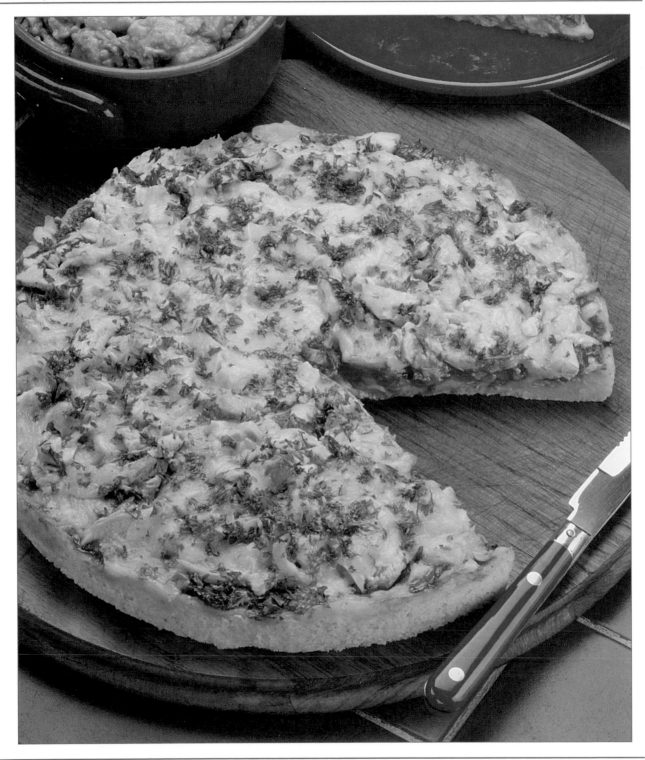

greek salad with dairy-free "feta"

dairy-free

dairy-free "feta"

- 1 package (about 14 ounces) firm or extra-firm tofu
- ½ cup extra virgin olive oil
- ¼ cup lemon juice
- 2 teaspoons salt
- 2 teaspoons Greek or Italian seasoning
- ½ teaspoon black pepper
- 1 teaspoon onion powder
- ½ teaspoon garlic powder

salad

- 1 pint grape tomatoes, halved
- 2 seedless cucumbers, sliced
- 1 yellow bell pepper, cut into slivers
- 1 small red onion, thinly sliced

1. Cut tofu crosswise into 2 pieces, each about 1-inch thick. Place on cutting board lined with paper towels; top with layer of paper towels. Place weighted baking dish on top of tofu. Let stand 30 minutes to drain. Pat tofu dry and crumble into large bowl.

2. Combine oil, lemon juice, salt, Greek seasoning and pepper in small jar with lid; shake to combine well. Reserve ¼ cup of mixture for salad dressing. Add onion powder and garlic powder to remaining mixture. Pour over tofu and toss gently. Refrigerate overnight or at least 2 hours.

3. Combine tomatoes, cucumbers, bell pepper and onion in serving bowl. Add tofu "feta" and reserved dressing. Toss gently.

Makes 4 to 6 servings

how-to

Why press tofu? It isn't absolutely necessary, but pressing removes excess moisture, which makes the tofu easier to handle and allows it to absorb flavors better. To press tofu, you need to make a sort of tofu sandwich. Place it on a cutting board or plate lined with a paper towels. Cover with more paper towels and place a flat, heavy object or objects on top. Press the tofu for 15 minutes or more. Keep an eye on the moisture that collects and drain it if needed.

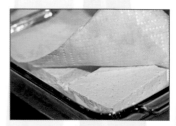

Press tofu between paper towels.

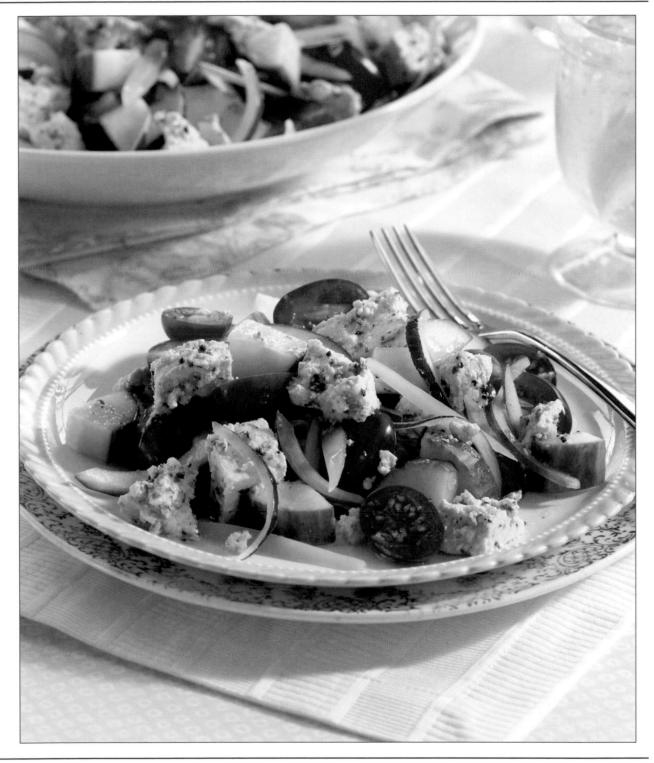

italian eggplant with millet & pepper stuffing

dairy-free

¼ cup uncooked millet
2 small eggplants (about ¾ pound)
¼ cup chopped red bell pepper, divided
¼ cup chopped green bell pepper, divided
1 teaspoon olive oil
1 clove garlic, minced
1½ cups vegetable broth
½ teaspoon ground cumin
½ teaspoon dried oregano
⅛ teaspoon red pepper flakes

1. Cook and stir millet in large heavy skillet over medium heat 5 minutes or until golden. Transfer to small bowl; set aside.

2. Cut eggplants lengthwise into halves. Scoop out flesh, leaving about ¼-inch-thick shell. Reserve shells; chop eggplant flesh. Combine 1 teaspoon red bell pepper and 1 teaspoon green bell pepper in small bowl; set aside.

3. Heat oil in same skillet over medium heat. Add chopped eggplant, remaining red and green bell pepper and garlic; cook and stir about 8 minutes or until eggplant is tender.

4. Stir in toasted millet, broth, cumin, oregano and red pepper flakes. Bring to a boil over high heat. Reduce heat to medium-low. Cook, covered, 35 minutes or until all liquid has been absorbed and millet is tender. Remove from heat; let stand, covered, 10 minutes.

5. Preheat oven to 350°F. Pour 1 cup water into 8-inch square baking pan. Fill eggplant shells with mixture. Sprinkle with reserved chopped bell peppers, pressing in lightly. Carefully place filled shells in prepared pan. Bake 15 minutes or until heated through.

Makes 4 servings

gluten-free info

Millet is an important grain in Asia, Africa and India, but probably most familiar here as an ingredient in birdseed. That's sure to change soon, because millet has a nut-like, mildly sweet flavor and is high in protein, minerals, vitamins and fiber. It is incredibly versatile and can be served as a cooked cereal, used as a side dish, added raw to baked goods for crunch, and even popped like popcorn for a snack.

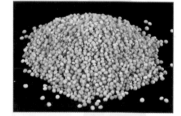

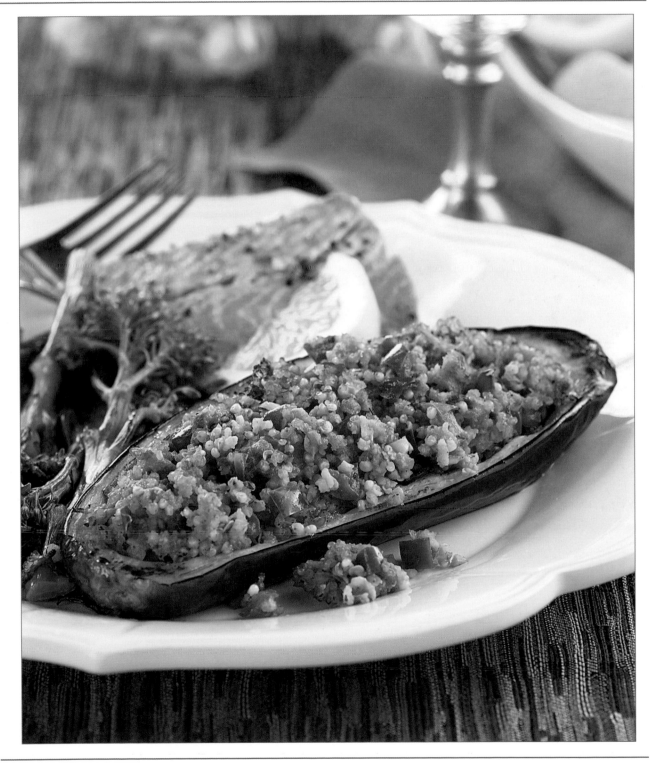

mediterranean vegetable bake

dairy-free

2 tomatoes, sliced

1 small red onion, sliced

1 medium zucchini, sliced

1 small eggplant, sliced

1 small yellow squash, sliced

1 large portobello mushroom, sliced

2 cloves garlic, finely chopped

3 tablespoons olive oil

2 teaspoons chopped fresh rosemary leaves

⅔ cup dry white wine

Salt and black pepper

1. Preheat oven to 350°F. Grease bottom of casserole or 13×9-inch baking dish.

2. Arrange slices of vegetables in rows, alternating different types and overlapping slices in pan to make attractive arrangement; sprinkle evenly with garlic. Combine olive oil and rosemary in small bowl; drizzle over vegetables.

3. Pour wine over vegetables; season with salt and pepper. Cover loosely with foil. Bake 20 minutes. Uncover; bake 10 to 15 minutes or until vegetables are tender. *Makes 4 to 6 servings*

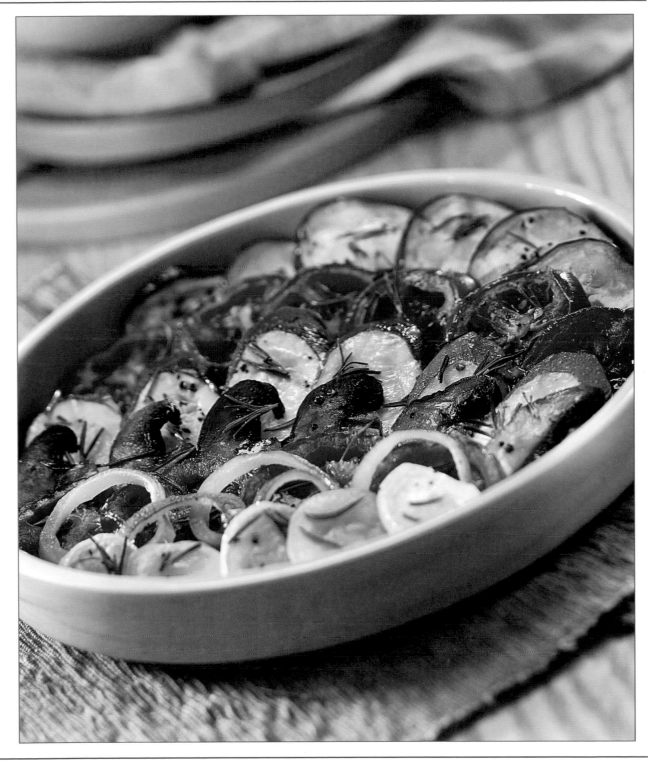

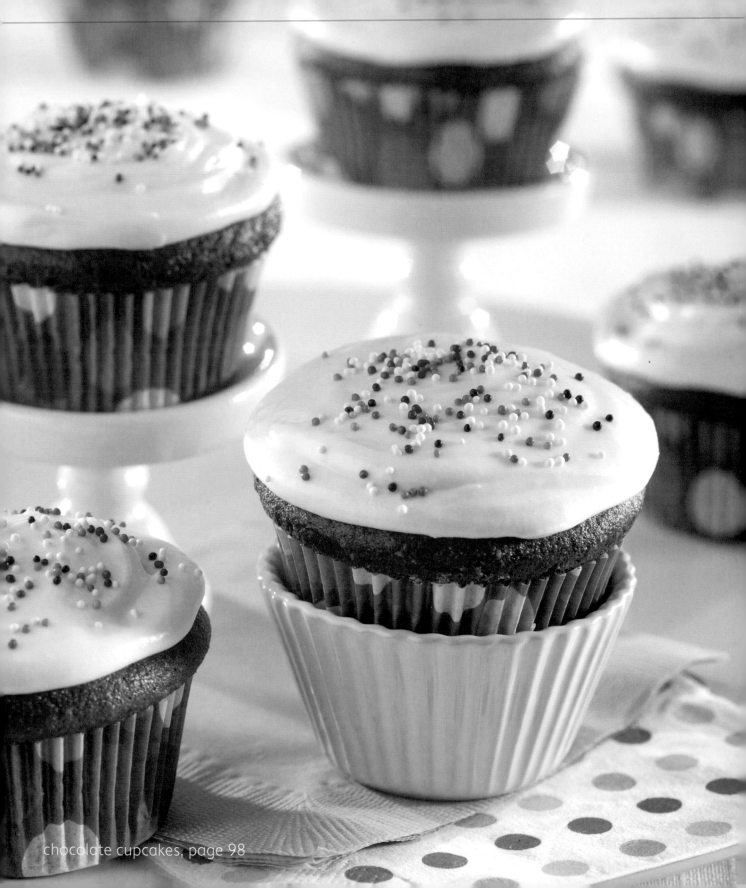

chocolate cupcakes, page 98

safe kid stuff

Birthday celebrations, after-school snacks, pizza parties—now your gluten-free kid can enjoy them all! Plenty of favorites, including brownies, pizza and layer cakes are here, plus new ideas like Mochi Rice Cake Rainbows and Kitty Cat Pancakes. Being gluten-free has never been more fun.

strawberry shortcake

2 pounds strawberries, sliced
½ cup sugar, divided
3 cups Gluten-Free All-Purpose Flour Blend (page 19)
4½ teaspoons baking powder
¾ teaspoon salt
¾ teaspoon xanthan gum
¾ cup (1½ sticks) cold butter, cut into pieces
1 to 1¼ cups half-and-half
1 tablespoon cinnamon-sugar (optional)
Whipped cream or whipped topping

1. Preheat oven to 400°F. Grease baking sheet or line with parchment paper. Combine strawberries and ¼ cup sugar in medium bowl. Mash slightly to release juices; refrigerate until ready to serve.

2. Combine flour blend, remaining ¼ cup sugar, baking powder, salt and xanthan gum in large bowl. Cut in butter with pastry blender or two knives until mixture resembles coarse crumbs. Add 1 cup half-and-half gradually, stirring with fork until rough dough forms. Add additional half-and-half by tablespoonfuls if needed.

3. Turn dough out onto floured surface. Pat into ¾-inch-thick layer. Cut dough with 2½-inch round biscuit cutter; place on prepared baking sheet. Pat remaining dough together and cut out additional biscuits. Brush tops with additional half-and-half and sprinkle with cinnamon-sugar, if desired.

4. Bake 15 to 20 minutes or until golden brown. Transfer to wire rack to cool. Split biscuits; top with strawberry mixture and whipped cream. *Makes 6 to 8 servings*

dairy-free variation

Replace butter with cold dairy-free stick margarine (not spread). Replace half-and-half with soy creamer. Omit whipped topping or top with dairy-free ice cream.

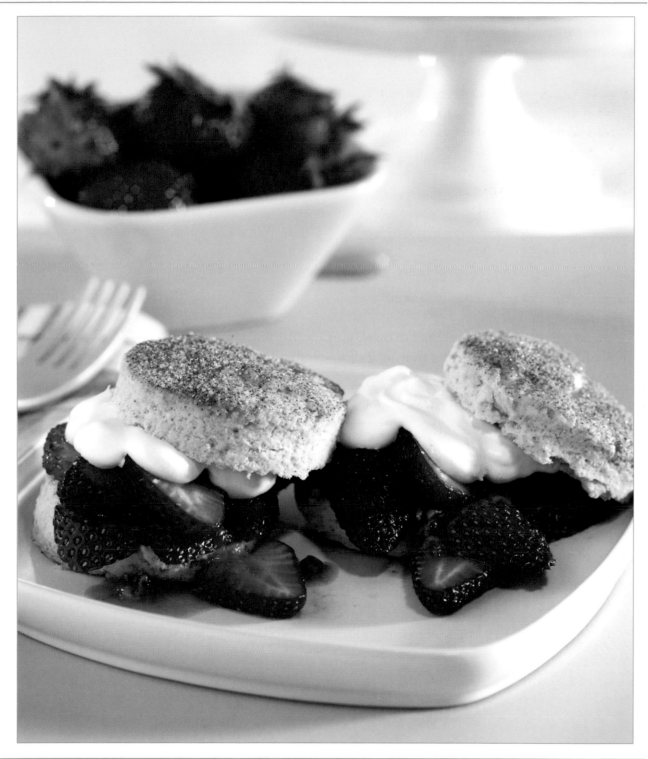

kids' pizzas

dairy-free

3 cups Gluten-Free Flour Blend for Breads (page 19)
2 packages (¼ ounce each) active dry yeast
2 teaspoons xanthan gum
1 teaspoon salt
1¼ cups warm water, divided
¼ cup extra virgin olive oil
3 egg whites
1 tablespoon honey
1 teaspoon cider vinegar

toppings

1 can (about 14 ounces) pizza sauce
Italian seasoning
1 package (about 3 ounces) sliced pepperoni
Shredded dairy-free cheese alternative (optional)

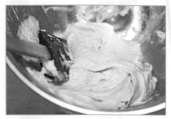
Dough should be smooth and thick.

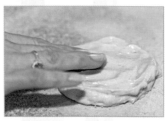
Pat dough out on prepared baking sheet with dampened fingers or oiled spoon.

1. Preheat oven to 450°F. Line baking sheet or pizza pans with parchment paper or sprinkle with cornmeal.

2. Mix flour blend, yeast, xanthan gum and salt in large bowl. Whisk 1 cup warm water, oil, egg whites, honey and vinegar together in medium bowl. Beat wet ingredients into dry ingredients with electric mixer at low speed until combined. Add additional water by tablespoonfuls until batter is smooth and thick. Beat 5 minutes on medium-high, scraping bowl occasionally.

3. Transfer one sixth of dough to prepared pan. Spread dough into 5- or 6-inch circle using dampened fingers or back of oiled spoon. Spread dough to desired thickness making crust thicker around edge to hold toppings. Repeat with remaining dough.

4. Bake 8 to 12 minutes or until crusts are lightly browned.* Top crusts with pizza sauce, Italian seasoning, pepperoni and cheese alternative, if desired. Bake 2 to 5 minutes or until cheese melts.

Makes 6 (5- to 6-inch) pizzas

To freeze pizza crusts for later use, allow them to cool, wrap well and store in the freezer for up to 3 months.

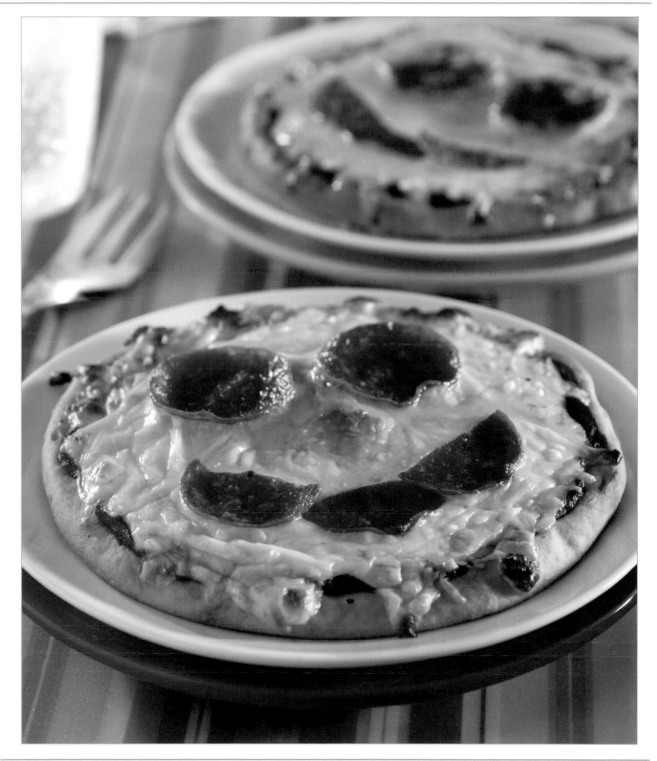

no-wheat brownies

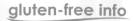
dairy-free

¼ **cup brown rice flour**

¼ **cup cornstarch**

1 **teaspoon baking soda**

¼ **teaspoon salt**

½ **cup (1 stick) dairy-free margarine**

1 **cup packed brown sugar**

½ **cup unsweetened cocoa powder**

½ **cup dairy-free semisweet chocolate chips**

1 **teaspoon vanilla**

2 **eggs, lightly beaten**

1. Preheat oven to 350°F. Spray 8-inch square baking pan with nonstick cooking spray. Combine rice flour, cornstarch, baking soda and salt in small bowl.

2. Melt margarine in large saucepan over low heat. Add brown sugar; cook and stir about 4 minutes or until sugar is completely dissolved and mixture is smooth. Remove from heat; sift in cocoa and stir until combined. Add flour mixture and stir until smooth. (Mixture will be thick.)

3. Stir in chocolate chips and vanilla. Beat in eggs until mixture is smooth. Spoon batter into prepared pan.

4. Bake 25 to 30 minutes or until toothpick inserted into center comes out almost clean.   *Makes 8 brownies*

gluten-free info

Surprise! No xanthan gum in this recipe. Because these brownies are so dense, it's not needed. Flourless Chocolate Cake (page 224), which has a similar texture, is also made without xanthan gum.

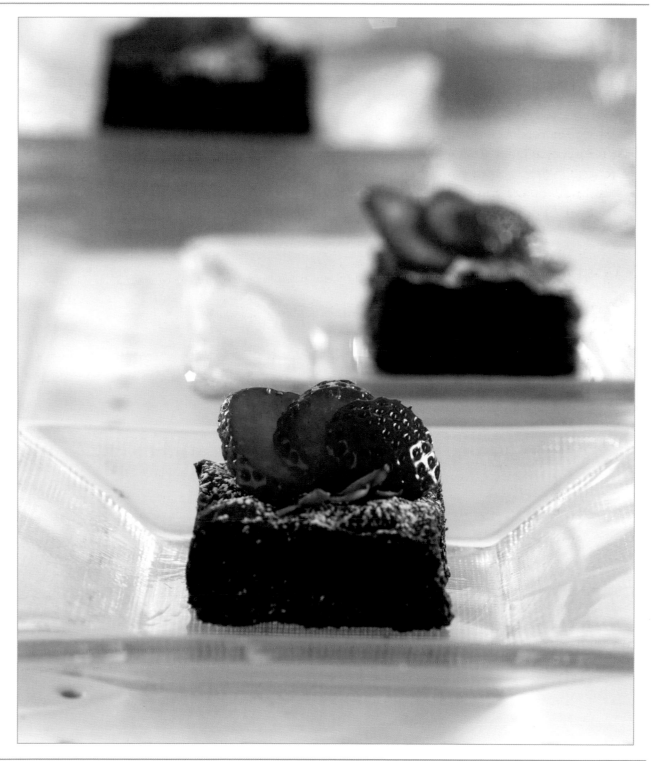

yam yums

2 large sweet potatoes, unpeeled, scrubbed
¼ cup maple syrup (not pancake syrup)
2 tablespoons orange juice
2 tablespoons butter, melted
⅛ teaspoon ground nutmeg
Salt and black pepper

1. Preheat oven to 350°F. Line baking sheet with foil.

2. Cut sweet potatoes crosswise into ½-inch-thick slices. Place slices on cutting board; use small metal cookie cutters (1½ inches in diameter) or sharp knife to cut shapes and letters from slices.

3. Combine maple syrup, orange juice and butter in small bowl. Arrange potato shapes in single layer on prepared baking sheet. Season both sides with nutmeg, salt and pepper. Brush both sides generously with maple syrup mixture.

4. Bake 20 to 30 minutes or until tender, turning once and basting with remaining maple mixture. *Makes about 4 servings*

recipe notes

Pure maple syrup seems expensive, but the reason is that it takes from 20 to 50 gallons of sap to make a single gallon of syrup. It has considerably more flavor than pancake syrup, which is usually nothing more than corn syrup with some maple extract added. There are even grades of pure maple syrup: Grade A is amber and mellow-flavored; grade B is darker and has a heartier flavor; grade C is very dark and robust.

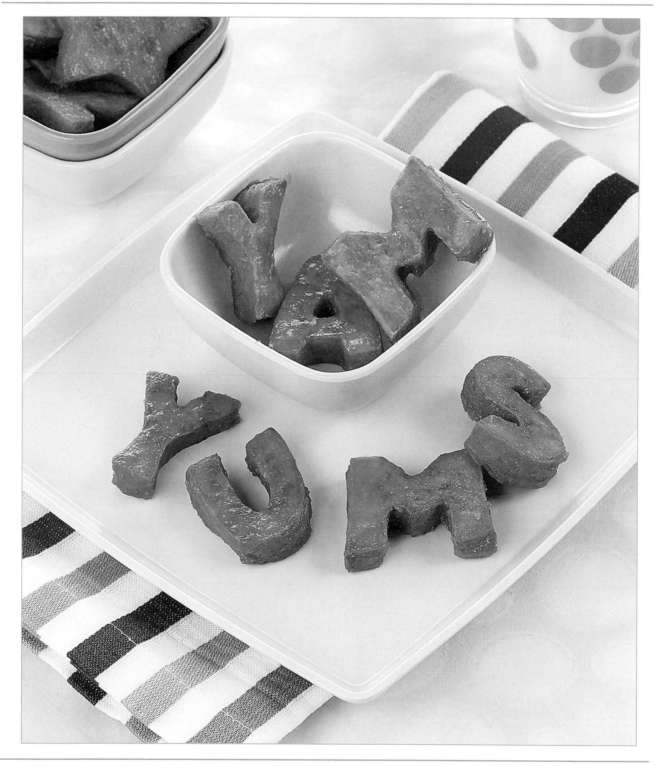

chocolate cupcakes

[pictured on page 88]

dairy-free

2½ cups Gluten-Free All-Purpose Flour Blend (page 19)

½ cup unsweetened cocoa powder

1½ teaspoons baking soda

¾ teaspoon xanthan gum

½ teaspoon baking powder

¼ teaspoon salt

1½ cups sugar

3 eggs

½ cup vegetable oil

1 teaspoon vanilla

1¼ cups plain soymilk, almond milk or other dairy-free milk

Creamy White Frosting (page 99)

1. Preheat oven to 350°F. Line 18 standard (2½-inch) muffin cups with paper baking cups.

2. Mix flour blend, cocoa, baking soda, xanthan gum, baking powder and salt in large bowl. Beat sugar, eggs, oil and vanilla in large bowl with electric mixer at medium speed 3 minutes or until thick and smooth.

3. Add flour mixture and soymilk alternately to sugar mixture, beating at low speed and scraping sides and bottom of bowl occasionally. Beat 2 minutes at medium speed.

4. Fill prepared muffin cups two-thirds full. Bake 20 to 25 minutes or until toothpick inserted into centers comes out clean. Cool on wire rack 5 minutes. Remove from pan; cool completely.

5. Meanwhile, prepare Creamy White Frosting; frost cupcakes.

Makes 18 cupcakes

creamy white frosting

dairy-free

4 ounces dairy-free cream cheese alternative, at room temperature

3 tablespoons dairy-free margarine, at room temperature

1½ teaspoons vanilla

4 to 5 cups powdered sugar

4 to 6 tablespoons plain soymilk, almond milk or other dairy-free milk

Beat cream cheese alternative and margarine in medium bowl until light and fluffy. Beat in vanilla. Gradually beat in sugar; add soymilk by tablespoonfuls until spreading consistency is reached.

giggle jiggles

dairy-free

2 cups pomegranate juice, divided

2 envelopes (¼ ounce each) unflavored gelatin

½ cup blueberries

1. Combine ½ cup juice and gelatin in small glass measuring cup. Let stand 5 minutes to soften.

2. Bring remaining 1½ cups juice to a boil in small saucepan. Stir in softened gelatin mixture until gelatin is dissolved.

3. Spray 8- or 9-inch square baking dish or pan lightly with nonstick cooking spray. Pour warm gelatin mixture into dish. Let cool to room temperature. Add blueberries. Refrigerate 3 hours or until firm.

4. Dip bottom of dish in warm water 15 seconds. Cut gelatin into small shapes with cookie cutters.* Lift shapes from pan. Reserve scraps for snacking or add them to a fruit cup.

5. Store in tightly covered container in refrigerator.

Makes 2 to 4 servings

Gelatin can be a choking hazard. Make sure children are seated and supervised while eating. Cut shapes into small bite-size pieces for younger children.

gingerbread people

½ cup (1 stick) butter, softened
½ cup packed brown sugar
⅓ cup molasses
1 egg
1 cup sorghum flour
1 cup white rice flour
¼ cup tapioca flour
2 teaspoons baking soda
1 teaspoon salt
1 teaspoon xanthan gum
1 teaspoon ground ginger
½ teaspoon ground allspice
½ teaspoon ground cinnamon
   Assorted gluten-free icings and/or candies

dairy-free variation

Replace butter
with dairy-free stick
margarine (not spread).
Decorate with dairy-free
icings and candies.

1. Beat butter and brown sugar in large bowl with electric mixer at medium speed until creamy. Add molasses and egg; beat until blended.

2. Combine sorghum flour, rice flour, tapioca flour, baking soda, salt, xanthan gum, ginger, allspice and cinnamon in large bowl. Whisk to combine.

3. Gradually add flour mixture to butter mixture, beating at low speed until dough forms. Shape dough into disc; wrap tightly in plastic wrap. Refrigerate 2 hours or until firm.

4. Preheat oven to 350°F. Grease cookie sheets. Roll out dough on lightly floured surface to ⅛-inch thickness. Cut out shapes with cookie cutter. Place cookies 2 inches apart on prepared cookie sheets.

5. Bake 10 to 15 minutes or until set. Remove to wire racks; cool completely. Decorate as desired. Store in airtight container.

Makes about 2 dozen cookies

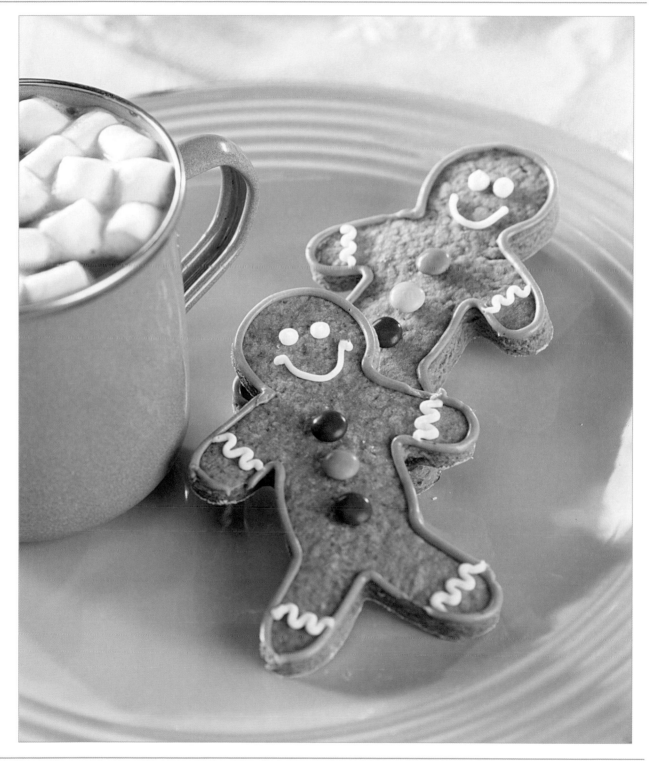

flourless fried chicken tenders

1½ cups chickpea flour (see sidebar)
1½ teaspoons Italian seasoning
  1 teaspoon salt
½ teaspoon black pepper
⅛ teaspoon ground red pepper
¾ cup plus 2 to 4 tablespoons water
  Oil for frying
  1 pound chicken tenders, cut in half if large
  Curry Mayo Dipping Sauce (see sidebar)

1. Sift chickpea flour into medium bowl. Stir in Italian seasoning, salt, black pepper and red pepper. Gradually whisk in ¾ cup water to make smooth batter. Whisk in additional water by tablespoons if needed until batter is consistency of heavy cream.

2. Meanwhile, add oil to large heavy skillet or Dutch oven to ¾-inch depth. Heat over medium-high heat until drop of batter placed in oil sizzles (350°F).

3. Pat chicken pieces dry. Dip pieces into batter with tongs; let excess fall back into bowl. Ease chicken gently into oil; fry 2 to 3 minutes per side until slightly browned and chicken is cooked through. Fry in batches; do not crowd pan.

4. Drain chicken on paper towels. Serve warm with Curry Mayo Dipping Sauce.   *Makes 4 servings*

curry mayo dipping sauce

Combine ½ cup mayonnaise, ¼ cup sour cream and ½ teaspoon curry powder in small bowl. Stir in 2 tablespoons minced fresh cilantro.

dairy-free variation

Prepare the dipping sauce with vegan (dairy-free, egg-free) mayonnaise or serve the chicken tenders with salsa or another dairy-free dipping sauce.

gluten-free info

Chickpea flour is also called garbanzo flour or besan flour. It is found in the specialty flour section of most supermarkets. It can also be purchased in Indian or Italian markets.

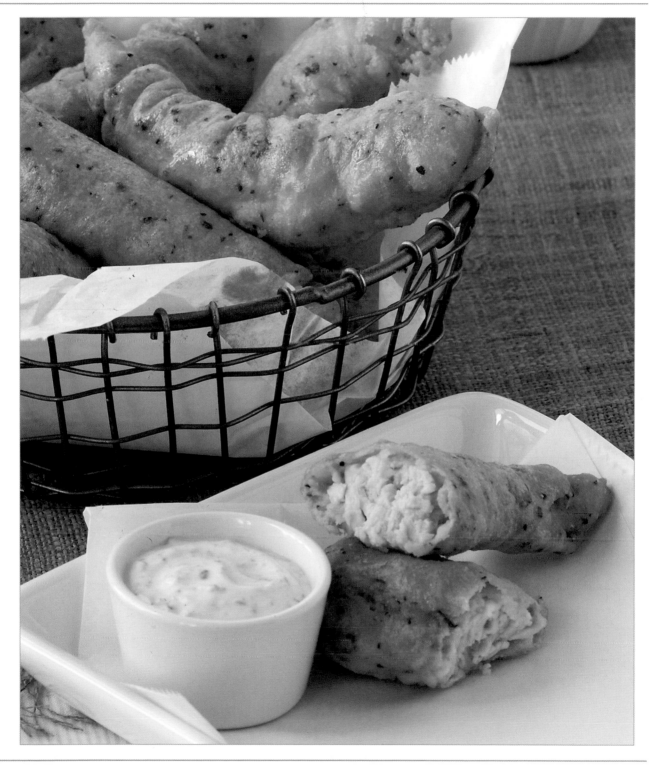

allergy-free birthday cake

dairy-free

allergy info

This delicious chocolate cake is not only gluten-free, it's also free from other common allergens. There are no eggs, dairy, wheat, tree nuts or peanuts. Soymilk can be replaced with another dairy-free milk to eliminate soy, another common allergen. Even kids with multiple sensitivities can enjoy a slice of this birthday cake.

3 cups Gluten-Free All-Purpose Flour Blend (page 19), plus extra for pans

2 cups sugar

6 tablespoons unsweetened cocoa powder

2 teaspoons baking soda

2 teaspoons xanthan gum

1 teaspoon salt

2 cups chocolate soymilk or other chocolate dairy-free milk

½ cup plus 2 tablespoons vegetable oil

2 tablespoons cider vinegar

1 teaspoon vanilla

No-Butter Buttercream Frosting (page 106)

1. Preheat oven to 350°F. Grease two 9-inch round cake pans with shortening or dairy-free margarine. Sprinkle with flour blend; tap out excess.

2. Whisk together flour blend, sugar, cocoa, baking soda, xanthan gum and salt in large bowl. Combine soymilk, oil, vinegar and vanilla in small bowl.

3. Pour wet ingredients into dry; stir thoroughly until smooth, scraping bottom and side of bowl. Immediately pour into prepared pans and place in oven.

4. Bake 25 to 30 minutes until toothpick inserted into centers comes out clean. (Middle of cake may look darker than edges.) Meanwhile, prepare frosting. Cool in pans 5 minutes. Carefully invert onto wire rack; cool completely.

5. Frost cake with No-Butter Buttercream Frosting. Decorate as desired. *Makes 10 servings*

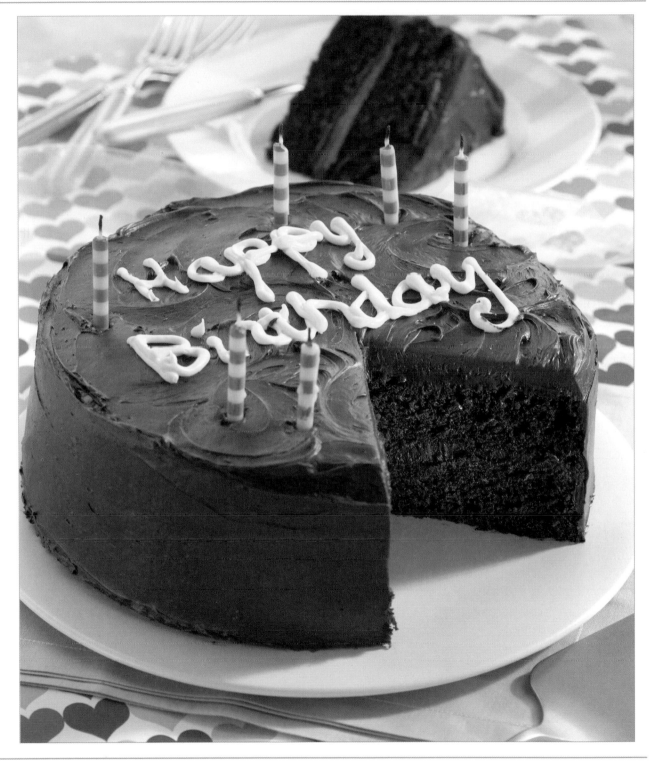

no-butter buttercream frosting

dairy-free

½ **cup (1 stick) dairy-free margarine (not spread)**
2 **teaspoons vanilla**
3 **to 4 cups powdered sugar**
½ **cup unsweetened cocoa powder**
4 **to 6 tablespoons soy creamer**

1. Beat margarine with electric mixer at medium speed until light and fluffy. Add vanilla.

2. Gradually beat in powdered sugar and cocoa powder; add soy creamer by tablespoonfuls until spreadable.

tickle sticks

dairy-free

1 **pound watermelon**
1 **container (6 ounces) dairy-free plain yogurt**
2 **teaspoons honey**
Grated peel and juice of 1 lime

1. Cut watermelon into 3×½-inch sticks. Remove and discard seeds.

2. Combine yogurt, honey, lime peel and lime juice in small bowl. Serve with watermelon sticks. *Makes 4 to 6 servings*

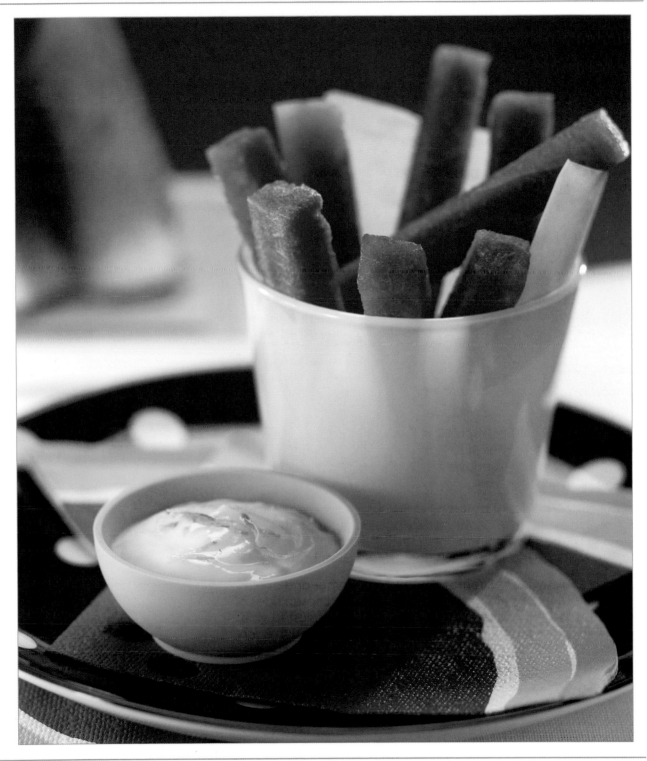

mochi rice cake rainbow

1 cup sweet rice flour (mochiko) (see sidebar)
¾ cup sugar
⅔ cup tapioca flour
   Pinch salt
1 can (13½ ounces) unsweetened coconut milk
¼ to ½ cup water
   Assorted paste food coloring

1. Spray 8×4-inch loaf pan or four 8-ounce custard cups with nonstick cooking spray. Set up steamer large enough to hold pan or cups over large saucepan of water.

2. Combine sweet rice flour, sugar, tapioca flour and salt in large bowl. Add coconut milk and whisk to combine. Whisk in water by tablespoons until batter is smooth with consistency of heavy cream.

3. Divide batter into 3 or 4 medium bowls or measuring cups. Add different food coloring to each bowl and whisk to blend completely. Bring water in saucepan to a boil.

4. Pour one layer of colored batter into prepared pan. (This color will be on top of finished mochi.) Place pan in steamer; cover and reduce heat to a simmer. Steam about 8 minutes or until mochi is set in center. Carefully uncover steamer and gently touch center of mochi to check doneness.

5. Pour second color of batter over first color. Layers can be as thick or thin as desired. Cover and steam 8 minutes or until second layer is set. Proceed with remaining batter, steaming each layer until set. Make as many layers as desired until all of batter is used.

6. When final layer is set, remove pan from steamer and cool. Refrigerate at least 1 hour or until ready to serve. Loosen sides of mochi from pan and invert onto serving dish. It is easiest to slice mochi with a plastic knife.   *Makes 6 to 8 servings*

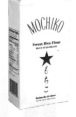

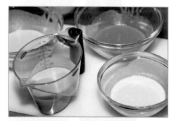

Divide batter into small containers and tint with food coloring.

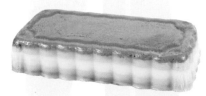

Let your child help choose his or her favorite colors for the rainbow.

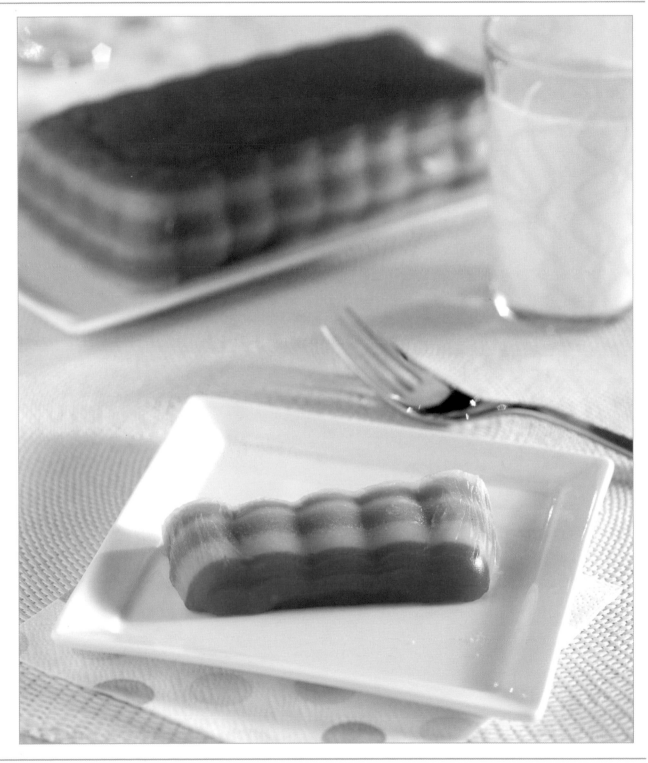

easy orange cake

 dairy-free

- 1½ **cups Gluten-Free All-Purpose Flour Blend (page 19)**
- ½ **cup sugar**
- 1 **teaspoon baking soda**
- 1 **teaspoon xanthan gum**
- ¼ **teaspoon salt**
- **Grated peel of 1 orange**
- ⅔ **cup orange juice**
- 5 **tablespoons vegetable oil**
- **Orange No-Butter Buttercream Frosting (recipe follows)**

1. Preheat oven to 350°F. Spray 8-inch square or 9-inch round cake pan with nonstick cooking spray.

2. Combine flour blend, sugar, baking soda, xanthan gum, salt and orange peel in medium bowl. Combine orange juice and oil in small bowl or measuring cup. Add wet ingredients to flour mixture and stir until smooth. Pour into prepared pan.

3. Bake 30 minutes or until toothpick inserted into center comes out clean. Meanwhile, prepare Orange No-Butter Buttercream Frosting. Cool cake 5 minutes in pan on wire rack; remove from pan and cool completely. Frost and decorate.   *Makes about 6 servings*

orange no-butter buttercream frosting

dairy-free

- ½ **cup (1 stick) dairy-free margarine (not spread)**
- 2 **teaspoons grated orange peel**
- 2 **tablespoons orange juice**
- 1 **teaspoon vanilla**
- 4 **cups powdered sugar**
- 4 to 6 **tablespoons soy creamer**

1. Beat margarine with electric mixer at medium speed until light and fluffy. Add orange peel, orange juice and vanilla.

2. Gradually beat in powdered sugar; beat in soy creamer by tablespoonfuls until spreadable.

Like the Allergy-Free Birthday Cake on page 104, this recipe is a gluten-free variation of an old recipe called Wacky Cake or Crazy Cake. Wacky Cake was supposedly invented either during the depression or World War II when ingredients like eggs and milk were hard to come by. Wacky Cake depends on an acid to activate the baking soda. In this recipe, orange juice is used. For Allergy-Free Chocolate Cake, cider vinegar is the acidic ingredient. Do NOT allow either cake to cool in the pan for more than 10 minutes or it can become gummy.

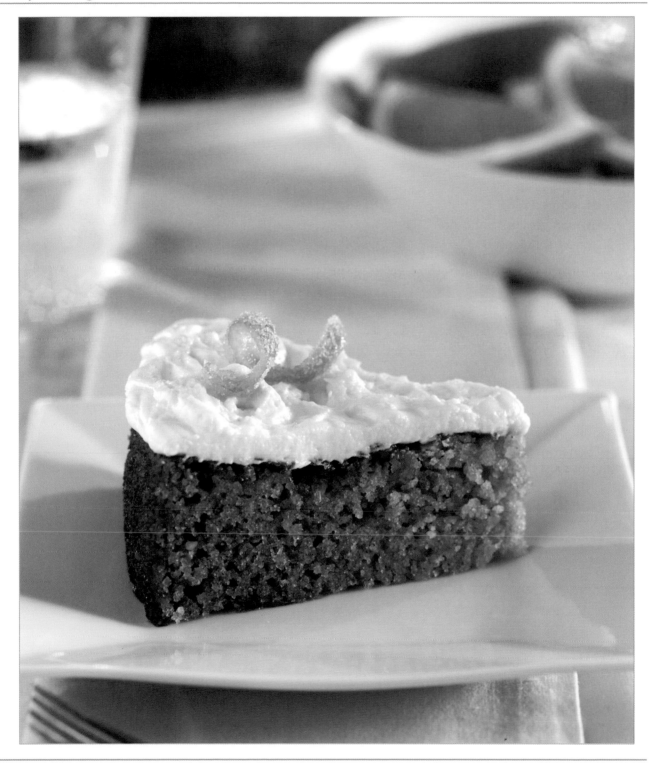

microwave chocolate pudding

 dairy-free

¼ **cup unsweetened cocoa powder**

2 **tablespoons cornstarch**

1½ **cups soymilk, almond milk or other dairy-free milk**

⅓ **cup sugar**

1 **teaspoon vanilla**

⅛ **teaspoon ground cinnamon**

Assorted sprinkles

1. Combine cocoa powder and cornstarch in medium microwavable bowl or 1-quart glass measure. Whisk in soymilk until well blended.

2. Microwave on HIGH 2 minutes; stir. Microwave on MEDIUM-HIGH (70%) 2½ to 4½ minutes or until thickened, stirring every 1½ minutes.

3. Stir in sugar, vanilla and cinnamon. Let stand at least 5 minutes before serving, stirring occasionally to prevent skin from forming. Spoon into serving dishes.

4. To serve cold, press plastic wrap onto surface of pudding to prevent skin from forming and refrigerate at least 1 hour. Garnish with sprinkles just before serving. *Makes 2 to 4 servings*

gluten-free info

Cornstarch is a fine, white powder made from the heart of corn kernels (the endosperm). It is used as a thickener in many recipes and products and also as an ingredient in many gluten-free flour blends. Don't confuse it with cornmeal or corn flour—unless you are in England where cornstarch is called corn flour!

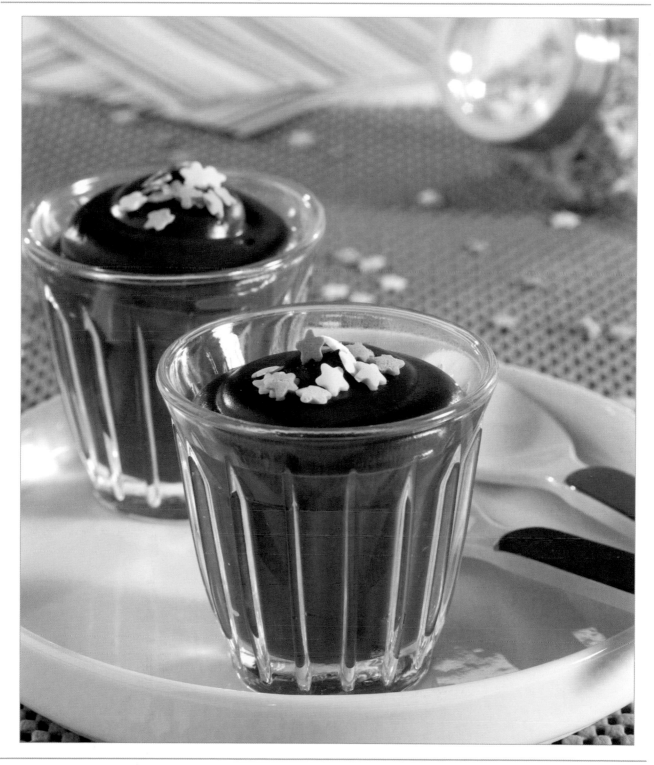

kitty cat pancakes

dairy-free

1¼ **cups rice flour**

¼ **cup tapioca flour**

¼ **cup cornstarch**

1 **tablespoon sugar**

1½ **teaspoons baking powder**

½ **teaspoon baking soda**

½ **teaspoon salt**

½ **teaspoon xanthan gum**

1 **cup plain soymilk, almond milk or other dairy-free milk**

2 **eggs**

3 **tablespoons vegetable oil**

Juice of ½ **lemon**

½ **teaspoon vanilla**

Decorations: dried cherries or raisins, thin slivers of red-skinned apple

1. Combine rice flour, tapioca flour, cornstarch, sugar, baking powder, baking soda, salt and xanthan gum in large bowl.

2. Stir in soymilk, eggs, oil, lemon juice and vanilla until thick batter forms. For thinner pancakes, add additional soymilk.

3. Lightly grease griddle or nonstick pan and heat over medium heat. Pour about ½ cup of batter on griddle. Spread batter to oval shape with back of spoon. Make kitty ears by spreading 2 points of batter upwards for ears, adding small amount of additional batter if needed.

4. Create eyes, nose and mouth by placing dried cherries or raisins gently on batter. For whiskers, place slivers of apple, peel side showing, onto batter. When surface of pancake becomes dull and bubbles appear (2 to 3 minutes), turn pancake. Cook 30 seconds to 1 minute or until lightly browned.

5. Repeat with remaining batter. Serve warm with maple syrup, if desired. *Makes about 8 pancakes*

variations

If you're not in the mood for kitty cats, this batter can also be poured into a circle and decorated with blueberries to make a smiley face. You can also create pancakes in the shape of letters or numbers. You probably have more ideas of your own!

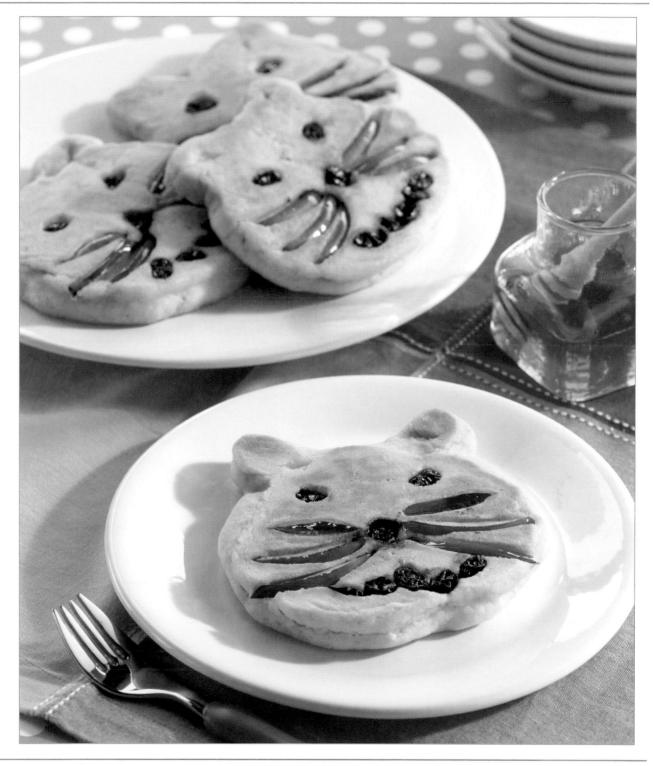

yellow layer cake

 dairy-free

2 cups Gluten-Free All-Purpose Flour Blend (page 19)

1¼ teaspoons baking powder

½ teaspoon salt

½ teaspoon xanthan gum

1¼ cups sugar

1 cup (2 sticks) dairy-free margarine

4 eggs

2 teaspoons vanilla

¼ cup soymilk, almond milk or other dairy-free milk

Dark Chocolate Frosting (page 118)

1. Preheat oven to 350°F. Spray two 9-inch round cake pans with nonstick cooking spray. Line bottoms with parchment paper or dust with flour blend.

2. Combine flour blend, baking powder, salt and xanthan gum in medium bowl.

3. Beat sugar and margarine in large bowl with electric mixer at medium speed 8 minutes or until light and fluffy. Add eggs, one at a time, beating well after each addition. Beat in vanilla.

4. Add flour mixture and soymilk alternately to sugar mixture, beating at low speed and scraping sides and bottom of bowl occasionally. Beat at medium speed 2 minutes.

5. Divide batter between prepared pans. Tap bottoms of pans on counter to even out batter. Bake 35 to 40 minutes or until toothpick inserted into centers comes out clean.

6. Cool 5 minutes in pans on wire rack. Remove from pans; cool completely.

7. Meanwhile, prepare Dark Chocolate Frosting. Frost cake.

Makes 10 servings

gluten-free info

It's best to bring all ingredients to room temperature when you're making gluten-free baked goods. Remove flour blends, butter or margarine and eggs from the refrigerator or freezer ahead of time. If you need to warm up the eggs because you forgot, place them in a bowl and cover them with warm tap water until needed.

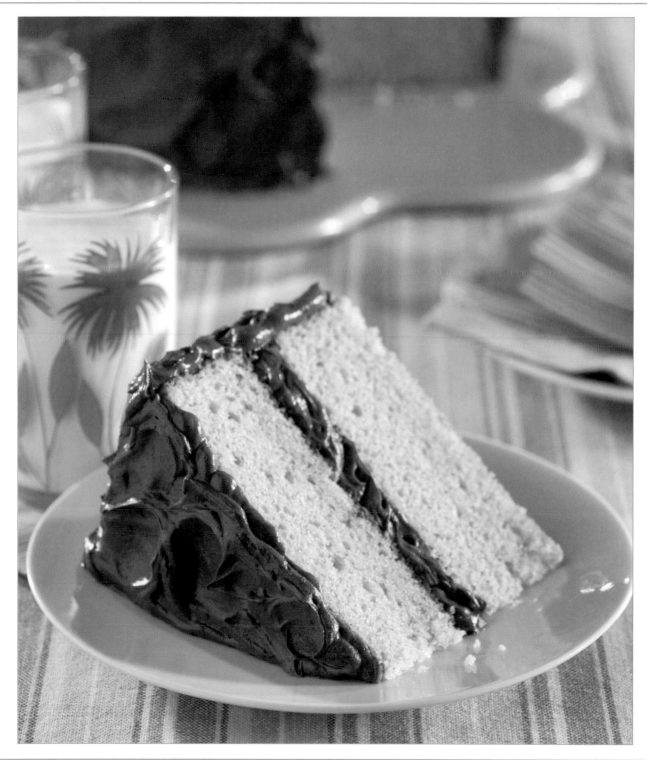

dark chocolate frosting

 dairy-free

- 1 cup (2 sticks) dairy-free margarine (not spread)
- 3 cups sifted powdered sugar
- 7 ounces dairy-free semisweet chocolate, melted
- ⅓ cup unsweetened cocoa powder
- ⅔ to 1 cup soy creamer
- 1½ teaspoons vanilla

1. Beat margarine in medium bowl until light and fluffy. Gradually beat in powdered sugar, alternately with melted chocolate and cocoa.

2. Beat in soy creamer by tablespoonfuls until spreadable. Beat in vanilla.

corny face

dairy-free variation

Replace cheese with dairy-free cheese alternative.

- Nonstick cooking spray
- 1 corn tortilla
- 1 slice provolone cheese *or* 3 tablespoons shredded Cheddar cheese
- ½ large dill pickle (cut lengthwise at an angle)
- 2 slices cucumber
- 2 pitted black olives
- 2 tablespoons shredded carrot

1. Lightly spray small skillet with cooking spray; heat over medium heat. Place tortilla in skillet; top with cheese. Heat 1 minute; fold tortilla in half to enclose cheese.

2. Cook tortilla 1 minute per side or until cheese is melted. Place tortilla on plate. Make face with vegetables.   *Makes 1 serving*

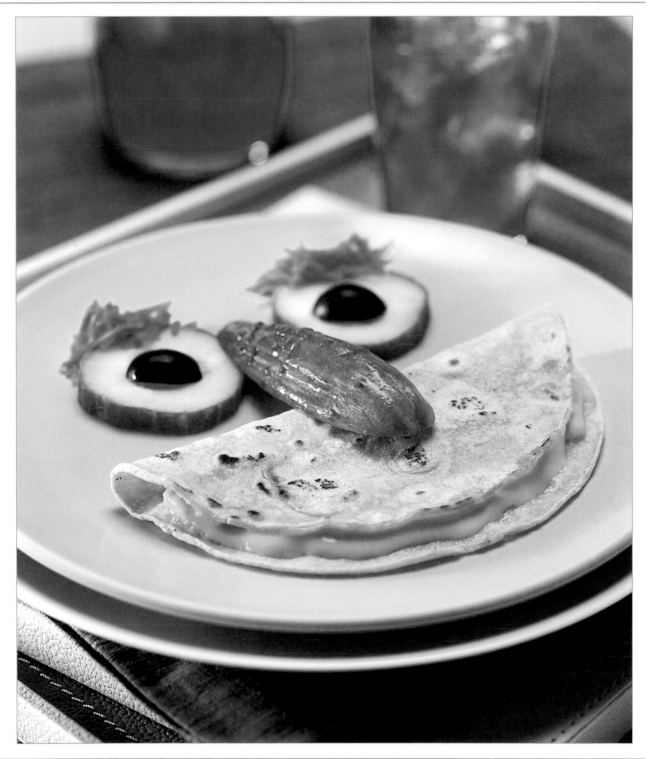

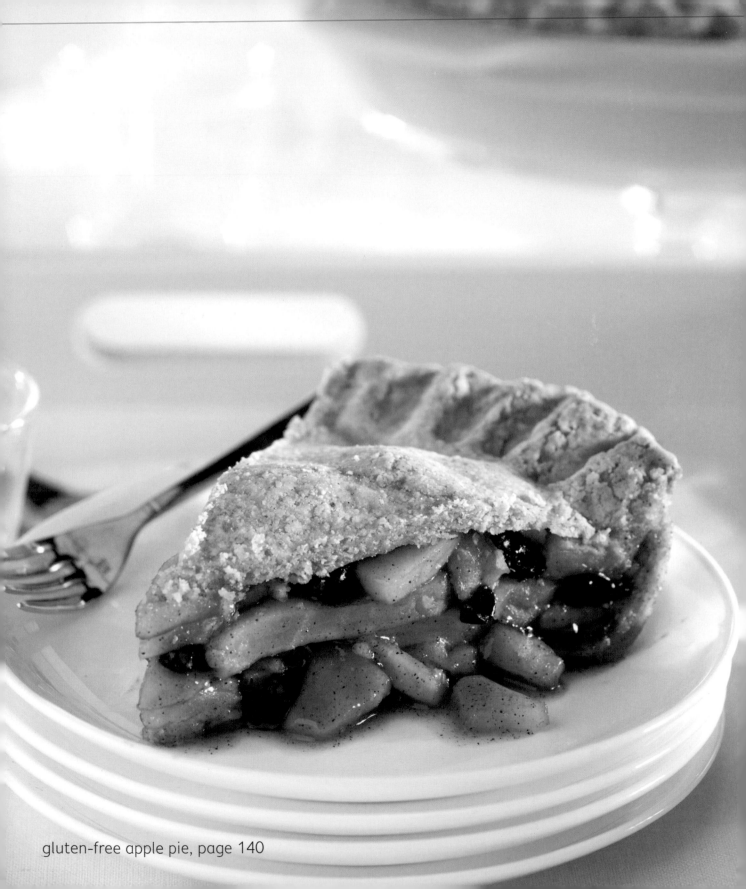

gluten-free apple pie, page 140

baking without

You don't have to give up your favorite baked goods or settle for less than delicious. With a few gluten-free flours and a little know-how, you'll be turning out fabulous Cinnamon Scones and Rosemary Bread in no time. Fill your kitchen with these wonderful aromas and the wheat won't be missed.

sandwich bread

 dairy-free

3 cups Gluten-Free Flour Blend for Breads (page 19), plus additional for pans

2 packages (¼ ounce each) active dry yeast

2 teaspoons xanthan gum

1 teaspoon salt

1 cup warm water, plus additional as needed

¼ cup vegetable oil

2 eggs, at room temperature

1 tablespoon honey

1 teaspoon cider vinegar

1. Line 9×5-inch loaf pan with foil, dull side out. (Do not use glass loaf pan.) Extend sides of foil 3 inches up from top of pan. Spray with nonstick cooking spray and sprinkle with flour blend.

2. Combine 3 cups flour blend, yeast, xanthan gum and salt in large bowl. Whisk 1 cup water, oil, eggs, honey and vinegar together in medium bowl. Beat into dry ingredients with electric mixer at low speed until batter is smooth, shiny and thick. Add more water by tablespoonfuls if needed. Beat at medium-high speed 5 minutes, scraping bowl occasionally.

3. Spoon batter into prepared pan. Cover with lightly oiled plastic wrap. Let rise in warm place 30 minutes or until batter reaches top of pan.

4. Preheat oven to 375°F. Bake 30 to 35 minutes or until bread sounds hollow when tapped and internal temperature is 200°F. Remove from pan and cool on wire rack. *Makes 1 loaf*

gluten-free info

Gluten-free breads generally need more yeast than conventional breads. The ideal temperature for rising is 80°F but monitor things closely. If the bread rises too quickly or rises over the top of the pan, it is more likely to fall after baking. If you do have a failure, don't give up and don't toss it out. Even funny looking bread usually tastes pretty good and any left over can easily be turned into gluten-free bread crumbs.

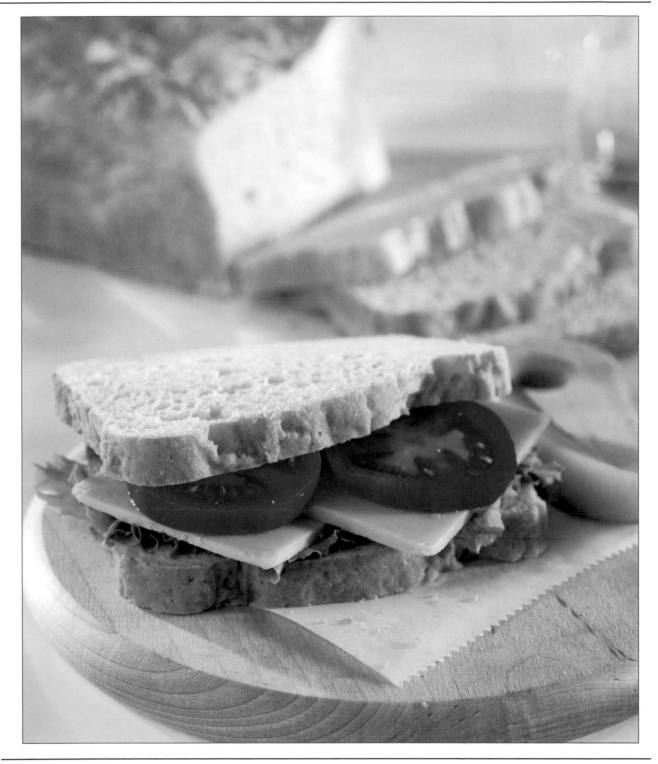

olive & herb focaccia

3 cups Gluten-Free Flour Blend for Breads (page 19)

2 packages (¼ ounce each) active dry yeast

2 teaspoons xanthan gum

1 teaspoon salt

1¼ cups warm water

¼ cup extra virgin olive oil

3 egg whites, at room temperature

1 tablespoon honey

1 teaspoon cider vinegar

toppings

1 cup chopped pitted kalamata olives

3 tablespoons chopped fresh rosemary leaves

2 tablespoons chopped fresh thyme

3 cloves garlic, minced

¼ cup extra virgin olive oil

Coarsely ground black pepper

¼ cup grated Romano cheese

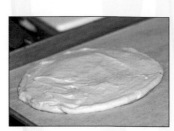
Let dough rest.

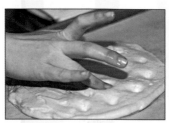
Dimple top of dough with fingers.

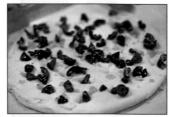
Sprinkle with toppings.

1. Combine flour blend, yeast, xanthan gum and salt in large bowl. Whisk 1 cup warm water, oil, egg whites, honey and vinegar in medium bowl. Beat wet ingredients into dry ingredients with electric mixer at low speed until combined. Batter should be smooth, shiny and thick. Add more water by tablespoonfuls, if needed. Beat at medium-high speed 5 minutes, scraping bowl occasionally.

2. Preheat oven to 450°F. Line large baking sheet with parchment paper or foil. Divide dough into two pieces; transfer to prepared sheet. Spread each piece into 8-inch round about ½ inch thick with dampened hands.

3. Let dough rest 20 minutes. Dimple top of dough with fingertips. Sprinkle with toppings; drizzle with oil and sprinkle with pepper.

4. Bake 15 minutes or until lightly browned. Sprinkle with cheese. Cool 3 minutes on wire rack before slicing.

Makes 2 focaccia breads

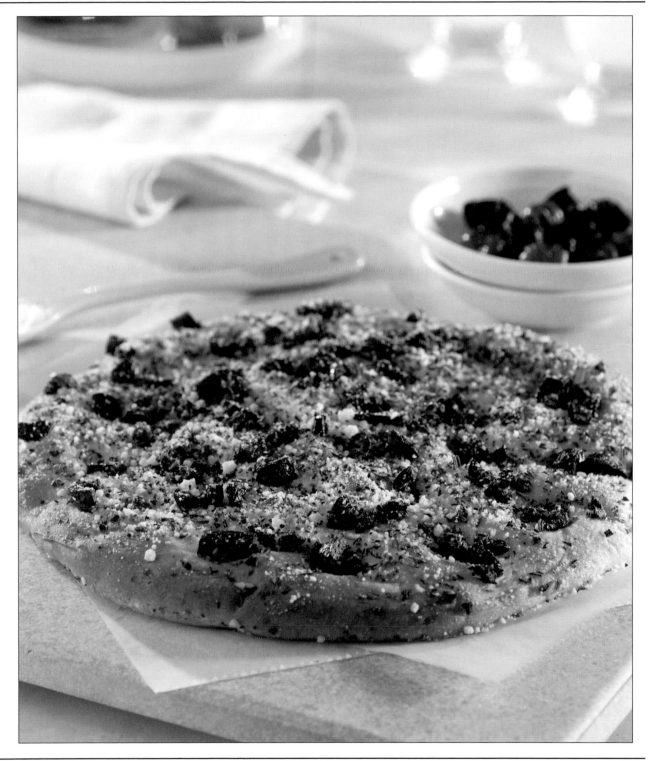

blueberry coconut flour muffins

   6 eggs
   ¼ cup (½ stick) butter, melted
   ¼ cup milk
   ½ cup sugar
   ½ cup plus 2 teaspoons coconut flour, divided (see sidebar)
   2 teaspoons grated lemon peel
   ½ teaspoon salt
   ½ teaspoon baking powder
   ½ teaspoon xanthan gum
   1 cup blueberries

1. Preheat oven to 375°F. Grease 12 standard (2¾-inch) muffin cups or line with paper liners.

2. Whisk eggs, butter, milk and sugar in medium bowl until well blended.

3. Thoroughly combine ½ cup coconut flour, lemon peel, salt, baking powder and xanthan gum in medium bowl. Sift flour mixture into egg mixture. Whisk until batter is smooth.

4. Combine blueberries with remaining 2 teaspoons coconut flour in small bowl. Stir gently into batter.

5. Fill prepared muffin cups almost full. Bake 12 to 15 minutes or until toothpick inserted into centers comes out clean. Cool 5 minutes in pan on wire rack. Remove from pan; serve warm.

Makes 12 muffins

dairy-free variation

Replace butter with dairy-free stick margarine (not spread). Replace milk with soymilk or other dairy-free milk.

gluten-free info

Coconut flour is a gluten-free, high-fiber, low-carbohydrate flour that adds a touch of sweetness to these muffins. Because it absorbs a great deal of liquid, a little coconut flour goes a long way. Most recipes using it also call for more eggs than usual, since it can become heavy without the extra lift that eggs provide. You will find coconut flour in the specialty flour section of many supermarkets. It can also be ordered on the Internet.

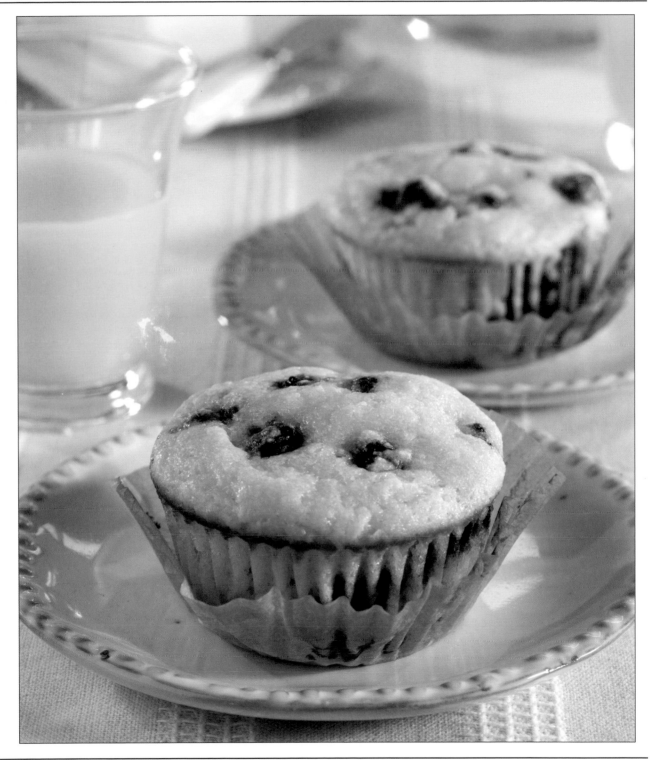

cinnamon raisin bread

- **3 cups Gluten-Free Flour Blend for Breads (page 19), plus additional for pan**
- **2 packages (¼ ounce each) active dry yeast**
- **2 teaspoons xanthan gum**
- **1 teaspoon salt**
- **1¼ cups plus 2 tablespoons warm milk, divided**
- **¼ cup vegetable oil**
- **2 eggs, at room temperature**
- **1 tablespoon honey or maple syrup**
- **1 teaspoon cider vinegar**
- **¾ cup raisins**
- **⅓ cup sugar**
- **1 tablespoon ground cinnamon**
- **1 tablespoon gluten-free oats (optional)**

1. Line 9×5-inch loaf pan with foil dull side out. (Do not use glass loaf pan.) Extend sides of foil 3 inches up from top of pan. Spray with nonstick cooking spray and sprinkle with flour blend.

2. Combine 3 cups flour blend, yeast, xanthan gum and salt in large bowl. Whisk 1¼ cups milk, oil, eggs, honey and vinegar in medium bowl. Beat milk mixture into dry ingredients with electric mixer at low speed until batter is smooth, shiny and thick. Beat at medium-high speed 5 minutes, scraping bowl occasionally. Stir in raisins.

3. Place large sheet of parchment paper on counter; sprinkle with flour blend. Scoop batter onto center of paper. Spread batter with back of oiled spatula or dampened hands to 9×18-inch rectangle ¾ inch thick. Brush remaining 2 tablespoons milk over dough. Combine sugar and cinnamon in small bowl. Sprinkle all but 1 tablespoon mixture over dough, leaving 1-inch border; lightly press into dough.

4. Using parchment, roll dough jelly-roll style beginning at short end. Push ends in to fit length of pan and trim excess parchment paper. Lift roll using parchment and place in prepared pan.

continued on page 130

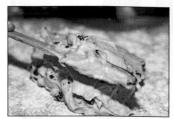

Scoop batter onto parchment paper.

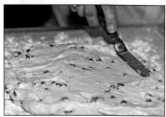

Spread batter with oiled spatula or dampened hands.

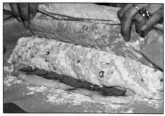

Roll dough beginning at short end.

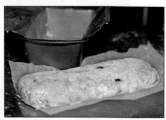

Ready to transfer to pan.

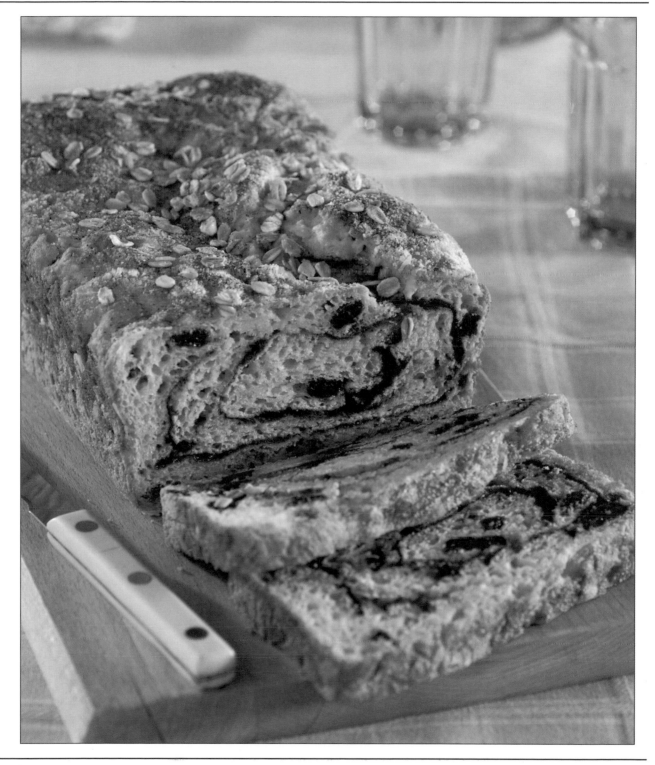

(Leave parchment in pan.) Sprinkle with remaining cinnamon-sugar and oats, if desired.

5. Cover loaf with lightly oiled plastic wrap; let rise in warm place 20 to 30 minutes or until batter reaches top of pan.

6. Meanwhile, preheat oven to 375°F. Bake 35 to 45 minutes or until bread sounds hollow when tapped and internal temperature is 200°F. Remove from pan; remove parchment and foil. Cool on wire rack.   *Makes 1 (9-inch) loaf*

brazilian cheese rolls (pão de queijo)

 1 cup whole milk
 ¼ cup (½ stick) butter, cut into pieces
 ¼ cup vegetable oil
 2 cups plus 2 tablespoons tapioca flour (see sidebar)
 2 eggs
 1 cup grated Parmesan cheese or other firm cheese

1. Preheat oven to 350°F.

2. Combine milk, butter and oil in large saucepan. Bring to a boil over medium heat, stirring to melt butter. Once mixture reaches a boil, remove from heat. Stir in tapioca flour. Mixture will be thick and stretchy.

3. Stir in eggs, one at a time, and cheese. Mixture will be very stiff. Cool mixture in pan until easy to handle.

4. Take heaping tablespoons of dough with tapioca-floured hands and roll into 1½-inch balls. Place 1 inch apart on baking sheet.

5. Bake 20 to 25 minutes or until puffed and golden. Serve warm.
                                    Makes about 20 rolls

gluten-free info

These moist, chewy rolls are a Brazilian specialty and are always made with tapioca flour instead of wheat flour. In Brazil they are popular at breakfast, lunch or dinner.

Tapioca flour can be found in most large supermarkets and is also readily available in Asian markets, where it is usually labeled tapioca starch. It comes from the cassava root (also called yuca or manioc), which is also the source of the tapioca used in puddings.

gluten-free lemon bars

1 cup Gluten-Free All-Purpose Flour Blend (page 19)
1 cup macadamia nuts or slivered almonds
½ cup (1 stick) cold butter, cut into pieces
½ cup powdered sugar
1 tablespoon plus 1 teaspoon grated lemon peel, divided
½ teaspoon salt
1 cup granulated sugar
3 eggs
⅓ cup lemon juice
Additional powdered sugar for dusting

1. Preheat oven to 350°F. Coat 9-inch square baking pan with nonstick cooking spray.

2. Place flour blend, nuts, butter, powdered sugar, 1 teaspoon lemon peel and salt in food processor. Process until mixture forms fine crumbs. Press mixture onto bottom of prepared pan. Bake 15 minutes or until light golden brown.

3. Beat granulated sugar, eggs, lemon juice and remaining 1 tablespoon lemon peel in large bowl with electric mixer at medium speed until blended.

4. Pour mixture evenly over warm crust. Bake 18 to 20 minutes or until center is set and edges are golden brown. Cool completely in pan on wire rack. Dust with additional powdered sugar. Store tightly covered at room temperature. *Makes 18 bars*

dairy-free variation

Replace butter with cold dairy-free stick margarine (not spread).

cinnamon scones

2 cups Gluten-Free All-Purpose Flour Blend (page 19), plus additional for work surface

¼ cup sugar

2½ teaspoons baking powder

¾ teaspoon salt

¾ teaspoon xanthan gum

½ teaspoon baking soda

⅓ cup cinnamon chips or chocolate chips

½ cup (1 stick) cold butter, cut into small pieces

¾ cup milk

½ cup plain yogurt

2 tablespoons cinnamon-sugar

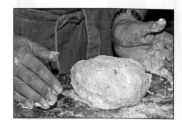

Transfer dough to floured surface. Knead 5 to 6 times.

1. Preheat oven to 425°F.

2. Combine flour blend, sugar, baking powder, salt, xanthan gum and baking soda in large bowl. Add cinnamon chips and toss to combine.

3. Cut butter into flour mixture with pastry blender or two knives until coarse crumbs form. Stir milk into yogurt in small bowl or large measuring cup until combined.

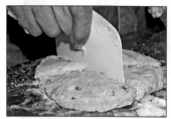

Divide dough in half.

4. Gradually add wet ingredients to dry ingredients, stirring just until dough begins to form. (You may not need all of yogurt mixture.) Transfer to surface sprinkled with flour blend. Knead 5 or 6 times until dough holds together. Divide into 2 pieces.

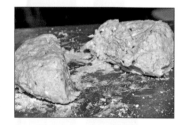

5. Pat each dough piece into 5-inch circle about ½-inch thick. Cut each circle into 6 wedges with floured knife. Place scones 2 inches apart on baking sheets. Sprinkle scones with cinnamon-sugar.

6. Bake 10 to 14 minutes or until lightly browned.

Makes 12 scones

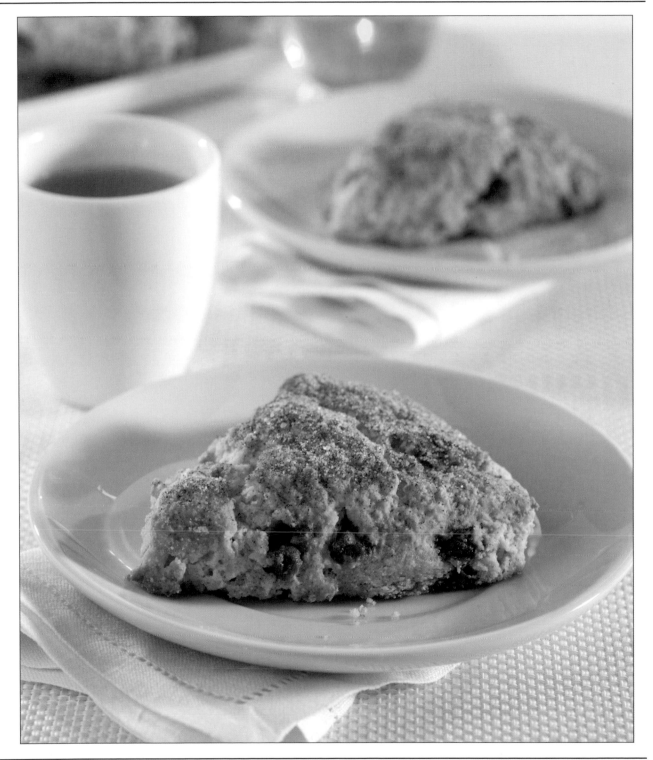

rosemary bread

2½ cups Gluten-Free Flour Blend for Breads (page 19), plus additional for pan

1 tablespoon active dry yeast (about 1½ packets)

1 tablespoon chopped fresh rosemary leaves

1½ teaspoon xanthan gum

1 teaspoon unflavored gelatin

½ teaspoon salt

2 eggs

¼ cup extra virgin olive oil

¾ cup warm milk (110°F)*

*Milk should be hot, but not over 120°F, which will kill yeast. Test temperature on inner wrist. Milk should feel warmer than body temperature, not burning hot.

1. Have all ingredients at room temperature. Spray 8×4-inch loaf pan with nonstick cooking spray and dust with flour blend.

2. Combine 2½ cups flour blend, yeast, rosemary, xanthan gum, gelatin and salt in large bowl. Beat eggs and olive oil in small bowl.

3. Beat egg mixture and milk into flour mixture with electric mixer at low speed until combined. Beat at high speed 3 to 4 minutes. Batter should be smooth and stretchy.

4. Spoon batter into prepared pan. Level top with dampened fingers or oiled spoon. Cover loosely; let rise in warm place about 45 minutes or until batter comes within 1 inch of top of pan.

5. Meanwhile, preheat oven to 400°F. Bake bread 10 minutes. *Reduce oven temperature to 350°F.* Cover bread loosely with foil. Bake 35 to 45 minutes or until bread sounds hollow when tapped and internal temperature is 190°F.

6. Remove bread from pan to wire rack; cool completely. Tightly wrap leftover bread and refrigerate up to 2 days. Freeze for longer storage.   *Makes 1 loaf*

gluten-free info

Several bread recipes in this book call for gelatin as an ingredient; it helps the structure and moisture of a loaf. Purchase plain, unflavored gelatin and measure out the correct amount from a packet. Fold the packet closed, clip it shut and store in a cool, dry area for the next use.

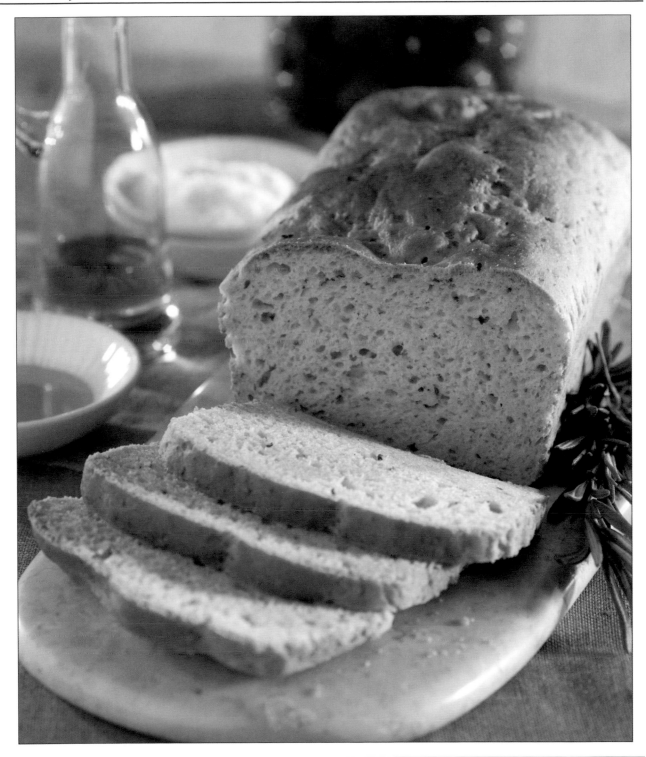

polenta apricot pudding cake

¼ **cup chopped dried apricots**

1½ **cups orange juice**

1 **cup ricotta cheese**

3 **tablespoons honey**

¾ **cup sugar**

⅔ **cup cornmeal**

½ **cup Gluten-Free All-Purpose Flour Blend (page 19)**

½ **teaspoon xanthan gum**

¼ **teaspoon ground nutmeg**

½ **cup slivered almonds**

1. Preheat oven to 325°F. Spray 10-inch nonstick springform pan with nonstick cooking spray.

2. Soak apricots in water in small bowl 15 minutes to soften. Drain and pat dry.

3. Beat orange juice, ricotta cheese and honey in medium bowl with electric mixer at medium speed 5 minutes or until smooth. Combine sugar, cornmeal, flour blend, xanthan gum and nutmeg in small bowl. Add dry ingredients to orange juice mixture; beat until combined. Stir in apricots.

4. Pour batter into prepared pan. Sprinkle with almonds. Bake 40 to 50 minutes or until center is almost set and cake is golden brown; serve warm. *Makes 8 servings*

gluten-free info

It's best to use a finely ground cornmeal in this recipe since the texture should be smooth. A coarse grind could cause grittiness. Always measure xanthan gum carefully for every recipe. Even ⅛ of a teaspoon more or less can make a difference.

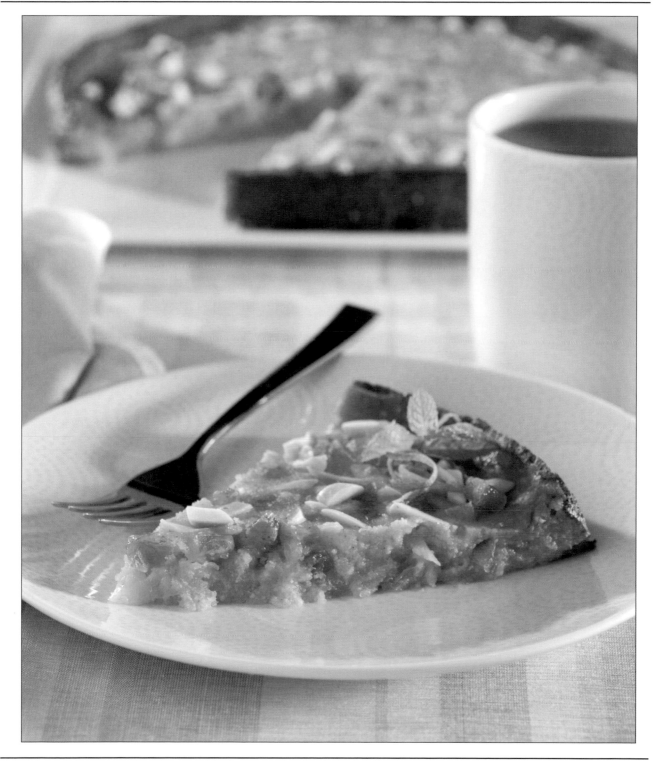

chili cheese bread

¾ **cup water**

2 **eggs**

3 **tablespoons olive oil**

1½ **cups Gluten-Free Flour Blend for Breads (page 19)**

1 **cup (4 ounces) shredded sharp Cheddar cheese**

1 **tablespoon sugar**

1 **tablespoon chili powder**

1 **package (¼ ounce) active dry yeast**

1½ **teaspoons xanthan gum**

1 **teaspoon unflavored gelatin**

½ **teaspoon salt**

1. Grease 8×4-inch loaf pan or spray with nonstick cooking spray.

2. Beat water, eggs and oil in large bowl with electric mixer at medium speed until combined. Whisk flour blend, cheese, sugar, chili powder, yeast, xanthan gum, gelatin and salt in large bowl until thoroughly mixed.

3. Gradually beat flour mixture into wet ingredients; beat at low speed 10 minutes. Batter will be sticky and stretchy. Spoon batter into prepared pan.

4. Cover; let rise in warm place about 1 hour or until dough almost reaches top of pan. Meanwhile, preheat oven to 350°F.

5. Bake 40 to 50 minutes or until bread sounds hollow when tapped and internal temperature is 190°F. Check after 20 minutes and cover with foil if bread is browning too quickly. Cool 10 minutes in pan on wire rack. Remove from pan; cool completely before slicing. *Makes 1 (8-inch) loaf*

gluten-free info

Several bread recipes in this book call for gelatin as an ingredient; it helps the structure and moisture of a loaf. Purchase plain unflavored gelatin and measure out the correct amount from a packet. Fold the packet closed, clip it shut and store it in a cool, dry place for the next use.

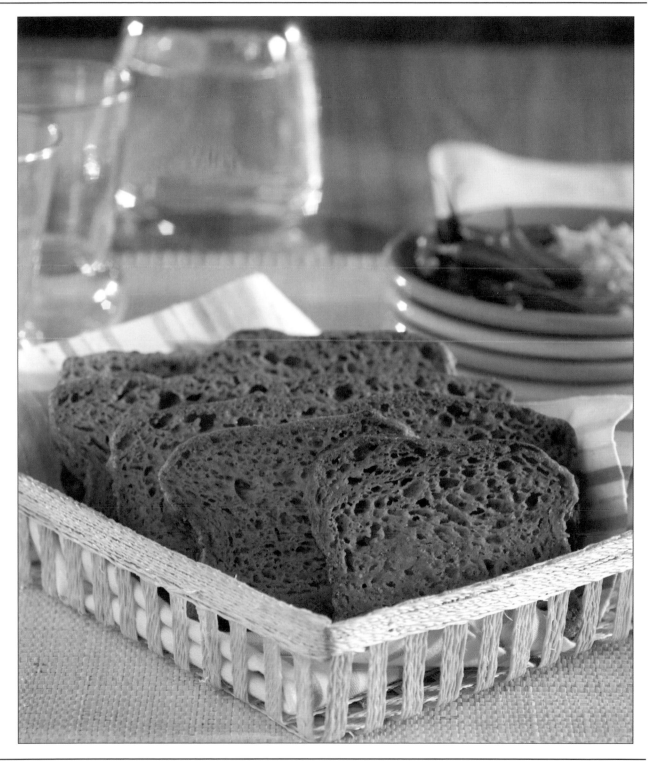

gluten-free apple pie

[pictured on page 120]

Gluten-Free Pie Crust (recipe follows)

6 tart apples, such as Gala, Jonathan or Granny Smith, peeled and cut into ¼-inch slices

¾ to 1 cup sugar, depending on sweetness of apples

½ cup dried cranberries

2 tablespoons cornstarch or tapioca flour

2 teaspoons lemon juice

1 teaspoon ground cinnamon

1. Prepare Gluten-Free Pie Crust. Generously butter 9-inch pie pan. Preheat oven to 425°F.

2. Combine apples, sugar, cranberries, cornstarch, lemon juice and cinnamon in large bowl; toss gently.

3. Press one crust into pan. Arrange apple mixture in crust. Place remaining crust over filling. Pinch edges of crust together; trim excess pastry. Cut slits in top of crust to vent steam.

4. Bake 12 minutes. *Reduce heat to 350°F.* Bake 30 to 40 minutes or until apples feel tender when pierced with tip of sharp knife. Cool on wire rack. *Makes 6 to 8 servings*

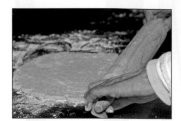

Roll out the dough.

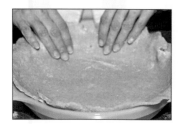

Place the crust in pie pan.

gluten-free pie crust

2 cups Gluten-Free All-Purpose Flour Blend (page 19)

¼ cup sweet rice flour

1 tablespoon sugar

1 teaspoon xanthan gum

½ teaspoon salt

¾ cup (1½ sticks) cold butter

2 eggs

1½ tablespoons cider vinegar

1. Mix flour blend, sweet rice flour, sugar, xanthan gum and salt in medium bowl. Cut in butter with pastry blender or two knives until mixture forms coarse crumbs.

2. Make a well in center of mixture. Add eggs and vinegar; stir together just until dough forms. Divide dough in half; shape into two flat discs. Refrigerate at least 45 minutes or until very cold.

3. Roll each piece of dough on floured surface to circle slightly larger than pie pan. (If dough becomes sticky, return to refrigerator until cold.) Refrigerate crusts in plastic wrap.

Makes 2 (9-inch) crusts

pink peppermint meringues

  3 egg whites
 ⅛ teaspoon peppermint extract
  5 drops red food coloring
 ½ cup superfine sugar*
  6 peppermint candies, finely crushed

*Or use ½ cup granulated sugar processed in food processor 1 minute until very fine.

1. Preheat oven to 200°F. Line cookie sheets with parchment paper.

2. Beat egg whites in medium bowl with electric mixer at medium-high speed 45 seconds or until frothy. Beat in peppermint extract and food coloring. Add sugar, 1 tablespoon at a time, while mixer is running. Beat until egg whites are stiff and glossy.

3. Drop meringue by teaspoonfuls into 1-inch mounds on prepared cookie sheets; sprinkle evenly with crushed candies.

4. Bake 2 hours or until meringues are dry when tapped. Transfer parchment paper with meringues to wire racks; cool completely.

Makes about 6 dozen meringues

gluten-free corn muffins

1 cup Gluten-Free All-Purpose Flour Blend (page 19)
1 cup cornmeal
½ cup sugar
1½ teaspoons baking powder
1 teaspoon baking soda
½ teaspoon salt
½ teaspoon xanthan gum
1 cup buttermilk
¼ cup (½ stick) butter, melted
2 eggs

1. Preheat oven to 350°F. Grease 12 standard (2¾-inch) muffin cups or line with paper baking cups.

2. Combine flour blend, cornmeal, sugar, baking powder, baking soda, salt and xanthan gum in large bowl. Whisk buttermilk, butter and eggs in medium bowl; stir into dry ingredients until well blended. Batter will be thick.

3. Spoon batter into prepared muffin cups filling almost to top. Bake 20 to 25 minutes or until lightly browned and toothpick inserted into centers comes out clean. Cool in pan 5 minutes; remove to wire rack. Serve warm.   *Makes 12 muffins*

dairy-free variation

A dairy-free alternative for buttermilk can be made by souring soymilk or other dairy-free milk. To make 1 cup, place 2 or 3 teaspoons of lemon juice or apple cider vinegar in a measuring cup. Add dairy-free milk to make 1 cup and set the mixture aside for 10 minutes before adding it to the recipe. Dairy-free margarine may be substituted for butter.

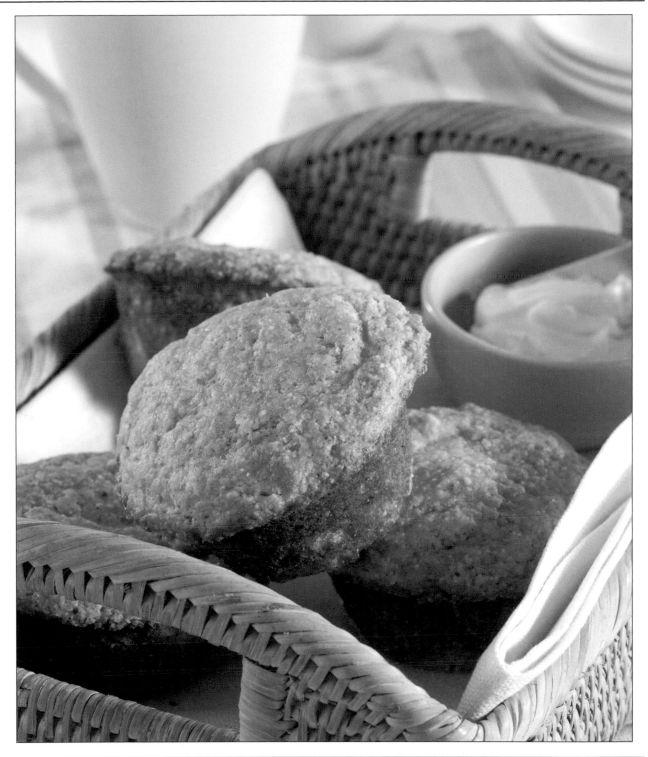

mini swirl cheesecakes

8 squares (1 ounce each) semisweet baking chocolate
3 packages (8 ounces each) cream cheese, softened
½ cup sugar
3 eggs
1 teaspoon vanilla

1. Preheat oven to 325°F. Lightly grease 12 standard (2¾-inch) muffin cups.

2. Place chocolate in 1-cup microwavable bowl. Microwave on HIGH 1 to 1½ minutes or until chocolate is melted, stirring after 1 minute. Let cool slightly.

3. Beat cream cheese and sugar in large bowl with electric mixer at medium speed about 2 minutes or until light and fluffy. Add eggs and vanilla; beat about 2 minutes or until well blended. Place 2 heaping tablespoons of mixture into each muffin cup.

4. Beat melted chocolate into remaining cream cheese mixture until well blended. Spoon chocolate mixture on top of plain mixture in muffin cups. Swirl batter together with knife.

5. Place muffin pan in larger baking pan; place on oven rack. Pour warm water into larger pan to depth of ½ to 1 inch. Bake cheesecakes 30 minutes or until edges are dry and centers are almost set. Remove muffin pan from water. Cool cheesecakes completely in muffin pan on wire rack.   *Makes 12 cheesecakes*

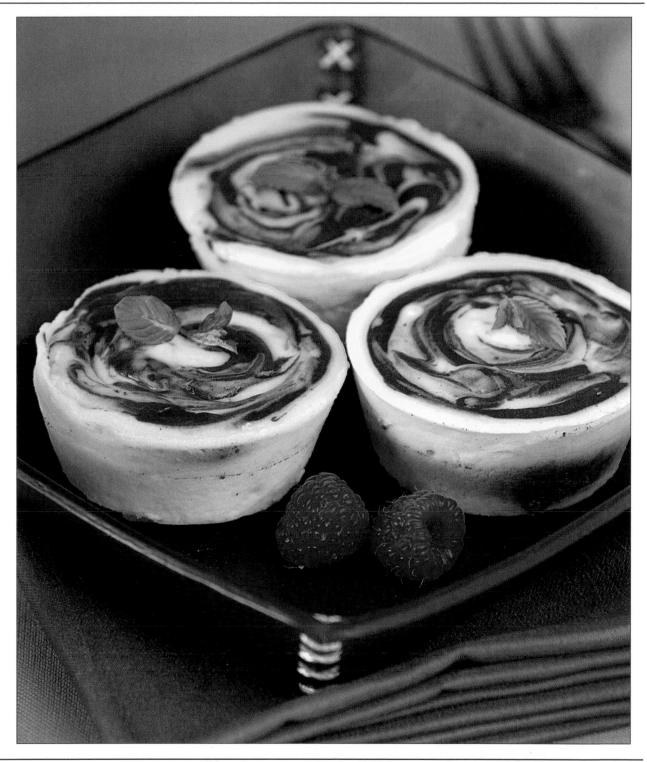

chili corn bread

Nonstick cooking spray
¼ cup chopped red bell pepper
¼ cup chopped green bell pepper
2 small jalapeño peppers,* minced
2 cloves garlic, minced
¾ cup corn
1½ cups yellow cornmeal
½ cup Gluten-Free All-Purpose Flour Blend (page 19)
2 tablespoons sugar
2 teaspoons baking powder
1½ teaspoons xanthan gum
½ teaspoon baking soda
½ teaspoon salt
½ teaspoon ground cumin
1½ cups buttermilk
1 egg
2 egg whites
¼ cup (½ stick) butter, melted

Jalapeño peppers can sting and irritate the skin, so wear rubber gloves when handling peppers and do not touch your eyes.

1. Preheat oven to 375°F. Spray 8-inch square baking pan with cooking spray.

2. Spray small skillet with cooking spray. Add bell peppers, jalapeños and garlic; cook and stir over medium heat 3 to 4 minutes or until peppers are tender. Stir in corn; cook 1 to 2 minutes. Remove from heat.

3. Combine cornmeal, flour blend, sugar, baking powder, xanthan gum, baking soda, salt and cumin in large bowl. Add buttermilk, egg, egg whites and butter; mix until blended. Stir in corn mixture. Pour batter into prepared pan.

4. Bake 25 to 30 minutes or until golden brown. Cool on wire rack.

Makes 12 servings

dairy-free variation

A dairy-free alternative for buttermilk can be made by souring soymilk or other dairy-free milk. To make 1½ cups, place 4 teaspoons of lemon juice or apple cider vinegar in a measuring cup. Add dairy-free milk to make 1½ cups and set the mixture aside for 10 minutes before adding it to the recipe. Dairy-free margarine may be substituted for butter.

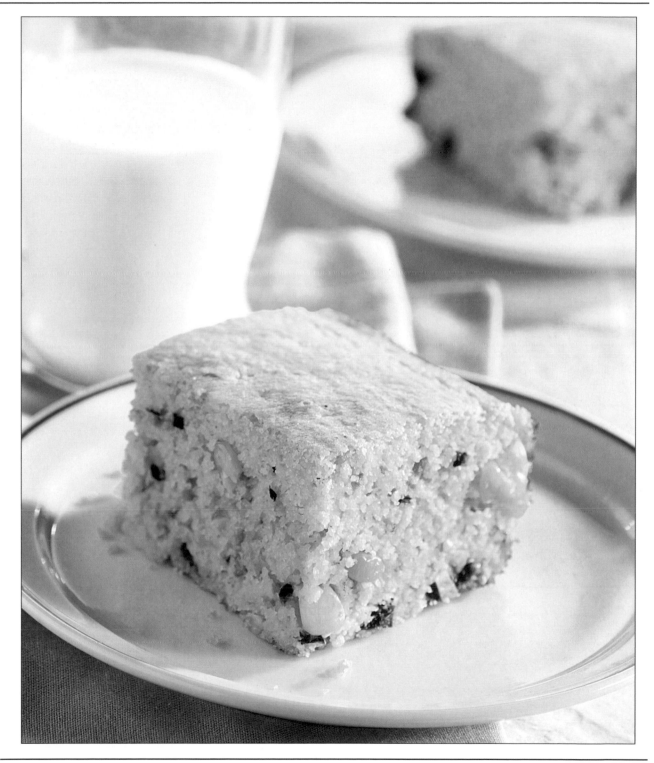

praline pumpkin pie

1½ **cups canned solid pack pumpkin**

½ **cup sugar**

½ **teaspoon salt**

1 **teaspoon ground cinnamon**

½ **teaspoon ground ginger**

½ **teaspoon ground cloves**

1½ **cups whipping cream**

2 **eggs**

4 **tablespoons unsweetened grated coconut, divided**

4 **tablespoons chopped pecans, divided**

1. Preheat oven to 425°F.

2. Stir together pumpkin, sugar, salt, cinnamon, ginger and cloves in medium bowl. Stir in cream and eggs until well blended.

3. Sprinkle 2 tablespoons coconut and 2 tablespoons pecans evenly over bottom of 9-inch pie pan. Pour pumpkin mixture into pan; spread evenly. Sprinkle with remaining coconut and pecans.

4. Bake 15 minutes. *Reduce oven temperature to 350°F.* Bake 40 to 50 minutes or until knife inserted into center comes out clean.

Makes 8 servings

gluten-free info

Using nuts and coconut for a gluten-free pie crust is a delicious workaround. If you prefer a more traditional pastry crust, try the Gluten-Free Pie Crust recipe on page 140.

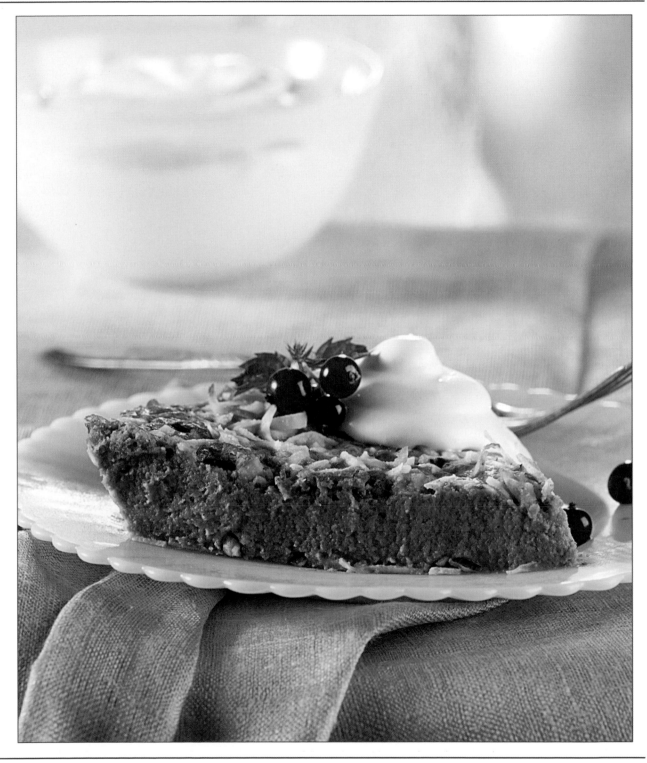

cellophane noodles with minced pork, page 154

hot & hearty

Whether you're getting a quick dinner on the table for the family on a weeknight or planning a fancy dinner party, you'll find the perfect entrée in this chapter. Choose from meat loaf, pizza, chicken, seafood or vegetarian recipes. There are tons of choices, every one of them without a speck of gluten.

southern fried catfish with hush puppies

   2 cups yellow cornmeal, divided
   ½ cup Gluten-Free All-Purpose Flour Blend (page 19)
   2 teaspoons baking powder
   2 teaspoons salt, divided
   ½ teaspoon xanthan gum
   1 cup milk
   1 small onion, minced
   1 egg, lightly beaten
   3 tablespoons white rice flour
   ¼ teaspoon ground red pepper
   4 catfish fillets (about 1½ pounds)
      Vegetable oil

1. Combine 1½ cups cornmeal, flour blend, baking powder,
½ teaspoon salt and xanthan gum in medium bowl. Stir in milk,
onion and egg until well blended. Let stand 5 to 10 minutes.

2. Combine remaining ½ cup cornmeal, rice flour, remaining
1½ teaspoons salt and red pepper in shallow dish. Coat both sides
of fish with cornmeal mixture. Heat 1 inch oil in large heavy skillet
over medium heat until 375°F on deep-fry thermometer.

3. Cook fish in batches 4 to 5 minutes or until golden brown and fish
begins to flake when tested with fork. Drain fish on paper towels.
Allow temperature of oil to return to 375°F between batches.

4. For hush puppies, drop batter by tablespoonfuls into 375°F oil.
Cook in batches 2 minutes or until golden brown. Drain on paper
towels.   *Makes 4 servings*

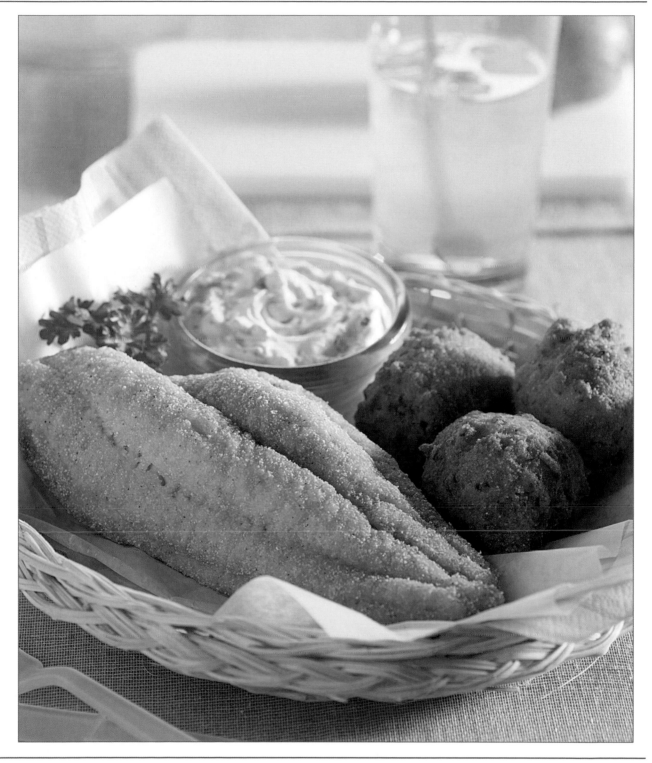

cellophane noodles with minced pork

dairy-free

[pictured on page 150]

 32 **dried shiitake mushrooms**
  1 **package (about 4 ounces) cellophane noodles (see sidebar)**
  2 **tablespoons minced fresh ginger**
  2 **tablespoons gluten-free black bean sauce (see sidebar)**
1½ **cups chicken broth**
  1 **tablespoon dry sherry**
  1 **tablespoon gluten-free soy sauce**
  2 **tablespoons vegetable oil**
  6 **ounces lean ground pork**
  3 **green onions, sliced**
  1 **jalapeño or other hot pepper, finely chopped**
    Chopped cilantro and hot red peppers (optional)

1. Place mushrooms in medium bowl; cover with hot water. Let soak 30 minutes or until softened. Squeeze out excess water. Discard stems; cut caps into thin slices.

2. Place noodles in medium bowl; cover with hot water. Let soak 15 minutes or until softened. Drain; cut into 4-inch pieces.

3. Combine ginger and black bean sauce in small bowl. Combine broth, sherry and soy sauce in medium bowl.

4. Heat oil in wok or large skillet over high heat. Add pork; stir-fry about 2 minutes or until no longer pink. Add green onions, jalapeño and black bean sauce mixture. Stir-fry 1 minute.

5. Add broth mixture, noodles and mushrooms. Simmer, uncovered, about 5 minutes or until most of liquid is absorbed. Garnish with cilantro and red peppers. *Makes 4 servings*

gluten-free info

Cellophane noodles are also called bean threads or glass noodles. They are thin, translucent noodles made from mung bean flour.

Chinese black bean sauce is made from fermented black soybeans (sometimes called salted or dried black beans). It is usually flavored with garlic, sugar and hot peppers. Although gluten-free black bean sauce is available, check labels carefully—most contain gluten in the form of soy sauce. You can also substitute actual fermented black beans, which are available in Chinese markets. For this recipe use 2 tablespoons of black beans and 1 tablespoon minced garlic.

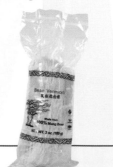

indian-style apricot chicken

dairy-free

6 skinless chicken thighs
¼ teaspoon salt
¼ teaspoon black pepper
1 tablespoon vegetable oil
1 large onion, chopped
2 tablespoons grated fresh ginger
2 cloves garlic, minced
½ teaspoon ground cinnamon
⅛ teaspoon ground allspice
1 can (14½ ounces) diced tomatoes, undrained
1 cup chicken broth
1 package (8 ounces) dried apricots
1 pinch saffron threads (optional)
Hot basmati rice

slow cooker directions

1. Coat 5-quart slow cooker with nonstick cooking spray. Season chicken with salt and pepper. Heat oil in large skillet over medium-high heat. Brown chicken on all sides. Transfer to slow cooker.

2. Add onion to skillet. Cook and stir 3 to 5 minutes or until translucent. Stir in ginger, garlic, cinnamon and allspice. Cook and stir 15 to 30 seconds or until mixture is fragrant. Add tomatoes and broth. Cook 2 to 3 minutes or until heated through. Pour into slow cooker. Add apricots and saffron, if desired.

3. Cover; cook on LOW 5 to 6 hours or on HIGH 3 to 3½ hours or until chicken is cooked through. Serve with basmati rice.

Makes 4 to 6 servings

how-to

To skin chicken easily, grasp the slippery skin with a paper towel and pull it away from the flesh. Repeat with a fresh paper towel as needed. Discard skins and towels. Wash your hands and work surfaces.

southwest spaghetti squash

1 spaghetti squash (about 3 pounds)
1 can (about 14 ounces) Mexican-style diced tomatoes
1 can (about 14 ounces) black beans, rinsed and drained
¾ cup (3 ounces) shredded Monterey Jack cheese, divided
¼ cup finely chopped fresh cilantro
1 teaspoon ground cumin
¼ teaspoon garlic salt
¼ teaspoon black pepper

1. Preheat oven to 350°F. Spray baking sheet and 1½-quart baking dish with nonstick cooking spray. Cut squash in half lengthwise. Remove and discard seeds. Place squash, cut side down, on prepared baking sheet. Bake 45 minutes or just until tender. Shred hot squash with fork; place in large bowl. (Use oven mitts to protect hands.)

2. Add tomatoes, beans, ½ cup cheese, cilantro, cumin, garlic salt and pepper; toss well. Spoon mixture into prepared baking dish. Sprinkle with remaining ¼ cup cheese.

3. Bake 30 to 35 minutes or until heated through. Serve immediately.

Makes 4 servings

how-to

To quickly cook spaghetti squash, cut the squash in half lengthwise. Remove and discard the seeds. Place, cut side down, in a microwavable baking dish. Add ½ cup water. Cover; cook on HIGH 10 to 15 minutes or until soft. Let cool 15 minutes. Scrape out squash "strands" with a fork. Makes about 4 cups cooked squash.

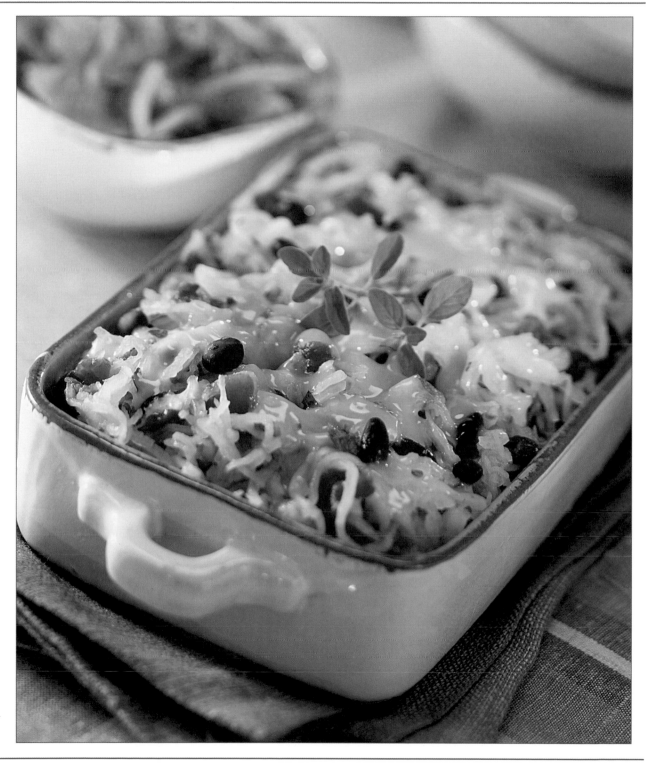

roast turkey breast with sausage & apple stuffing

- **8 ounces bulk pork sausage**
- **1 medium apple, peeled and finely chopped**
- **1 shallot or small onion, finely chopped**
- **1 stalk celery, finely chopped**
- **¼ cup chopped hazelnuts**
- **½ teaspoon rubbed sage, divided**
- **½ teaspoon salt, divided**
- **½ teaspoon black pepper, divided**
- **1 tablespoon butter, softened**
- **1 whole boneless turkey breast (4½ to 5 pounds), thawed if frozen**
- **4 to 6 fresh sage leaves (optional)**
- **1 cup chicken broth**

1. Preheat oven to 325°F. Crumble sausage into large skillet. Add apple, shallot and celery; cook and stir over medium-high heat until sausage is cooked through and apple and vegetables are tender. Drain fat. Stir in hazelnuts, ¼ teaspoon each sage, salt and pepper. Spoon stuffing into shallow roasting pan.

2. Combine butter and remaining ¼ teaspoon each sage, salt and pepper. Spread over turkey breast skin. (Arrange sage leaves under skin, if desired.) Place rack on top of stuffing. Place turkey, skin side down, on rack. Pour broth into pan.

3. Roast 45 minutes. Remove from oven; turn skin side up. Baste with broth. Return to oven; roast 1 hour or until meat thermometer registers 165°F. Let turkey rest 10 minutes before carving.

Makes 6 servings

dairy-free variation

Replace butter with dairy-free margarine or olive oil.

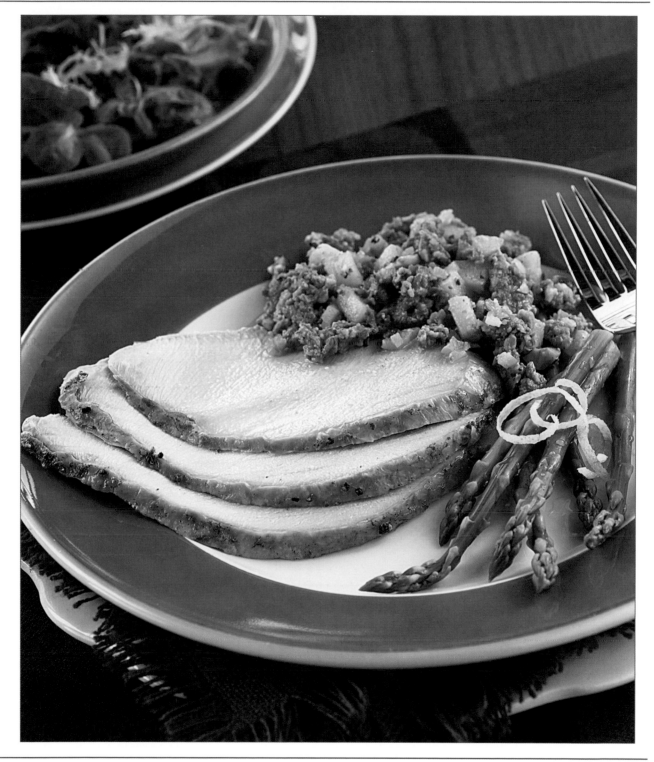

tuna steaks with tomatoes & olives

 dairy-free

1 tablespoon olive oil

1 onion, quartered and sliced

1 clove garlic, minced

1½ cups chopped tomatoes

¼ cup sliced pitted black olives

2 anchovy fillets, finely chopped (optional)

2 tablespoons chopped fresh basil

½ teaspoon salt, divided

¼ teaspoon red pepper flakes

4 tuna steaks (¾ inch thick)

Black pepper

Nonstick cooking spray

¼ cup toasted pine nuts (see sidebar)

1. Heat oil in large skillet over medium heat. Add onion; cook and stir 4 minutes or until translucent. Add garlic; cook and stir 30 seconds. Add tomatoes; cook 3 minutes, stirring occasionally. Stir in olives, anchovies, if desired, basil, ¼ teaspoon salt and red pepper flakes. Cook 8 to 10 minutes or until most of liquid evaporates.

2. Sprinkle tuna with remaining ¼ teaspoon salt and black pepper. Spray large nonstick skillet with cooking spray; heat over medium-high heat. Cook tuna 2 minutes per side or until medium-rare or desired degree of doneness. Serve with tomato mixture. Sprinkle with pine nuts.

Makes 4 servings

how-to

To toast pine nuts, place them in a small, dry skillet over medium-low heat. Cook, stirring occasionally, 3 to 5 minutes or until the nuts are fragrant and golden. Watch closely since pine nuts scorch easily.

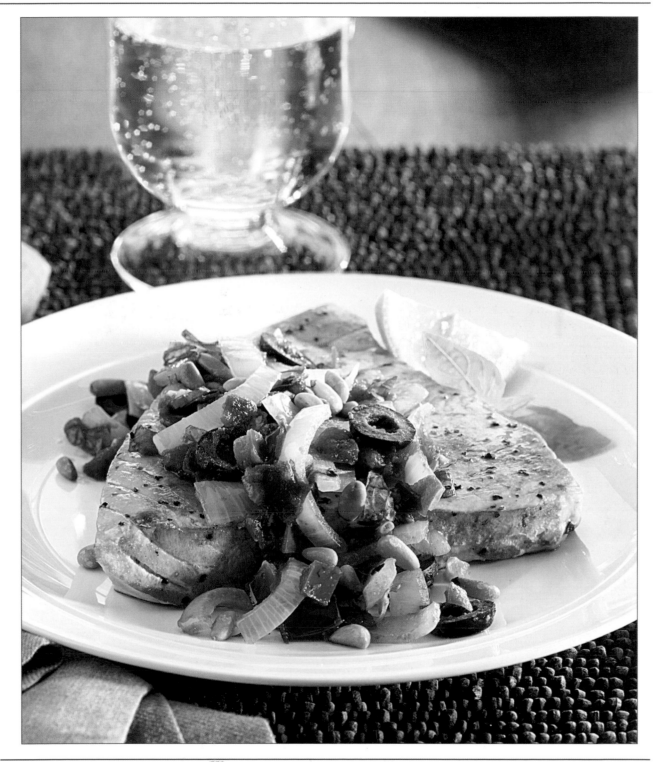

gluten-free pizza

1¾ cups Gluten-Free Flour Blend for Breads (page 19)

1½ cups white rice flour

2 teaspoons sugar

1 package (¼ ounce) active dry yeast

1½ teaspoons salt

1½ teaspoons Italian seasoning

1 teaspoon baking powder

½ teaspoon xanthan gum

1¼ cups warm water (110°F)

2 tablespoons olive oil

Pizza sauce

Toppings: fresh mozzarella, sliced tomatoes, fresh basil, grated Parmesan cheese

1. Combine all dry ingredients in large bowl. Add water in steady stream while beating with electric mixer at low speed until soft dough ball forms. Add olive oil; beat 2 minutes. Transfer to rice-floured surface and knead 2 minutes or until dough holds together in a smooth ball.

2. Place dough in oiled bowl; turn to coat. Cover; let rise 30 minutes in warm place. (Dough will increase in size but not double.)

3. Preheat oven to 400°F. Line pizza pan or baking sheet with foil. Punch down dough and transfer to center of prepared pan. Spread dough as thin as possible (about ⅛ inch thick) using dampened hands. Bake 5 to 7 minutes or until crust begins to color. (Crust may crack in spots.)

4. Spread pizza sauce over crust; sprinkle with toppings. Bake 10 to 15 minutes or until cheese is melted and pizza is cooked through.

Makes 4 to 6 servings

dairy-free variation

Omit the mozzarella and Parmesan cheeses or substitute a dairy-free cheese alternative.

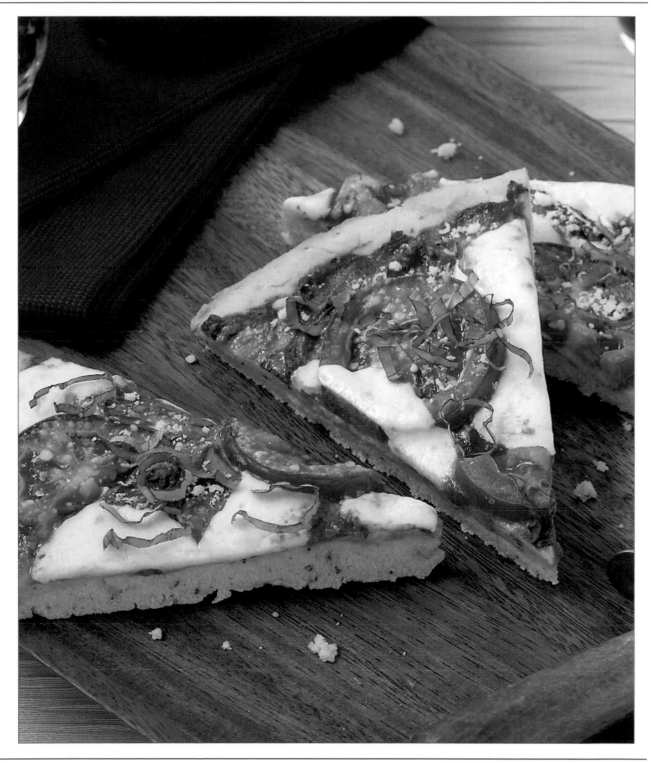

bean ragoût with cilantro-cornmeal dumplings

1 tablespoon vegetable oil

2 large onions, chopped

1 poblano chile, seeded and chopped

3 cloves garlic, minced

3 tablespoons chili powder

2 teaspoons ground cumin

1 teaspoon dried oregano

1 can (28 ounces) whole tomatoes, undrained, chopped

2 small zucchini, cut into ½-inch pieces

2 cups chopped red bell peppers

1 can (about 15 ounces) pinto beans, rinsed and drained

1 can (about 15 ounces) black beans, rinsed and drained

¾ teaspoon salt, divided

Black pepper

½ cup Gluten-Free All-Purpose Flour Blend (page 19)

½ cup cornmeal

1 teaspoon baking powder

¼ teaspoon xanthan gum

2 tablespoons shortening

¼ cup (1 ounce) shredded Cheddar cheese

1 tablespoon minced fresh cilantro

½ cup milk

1. Heat oil in Dutch oven over medium heat. Add onions; cook and stir 5 minutes or until tender. Add poblano, garlic, chili powder, cumin and oregano; cook and stir 1 to 2 minutes.

2. Add tomatoes, zucchini, bell peppers, beans and ¼ teaspoon salt; bring to a boil. Reduce heat to medium-low. Simmer, uncovered, 5 to 10 minutes or until zucchini is tender. Season with black pepper.

continued on page 166

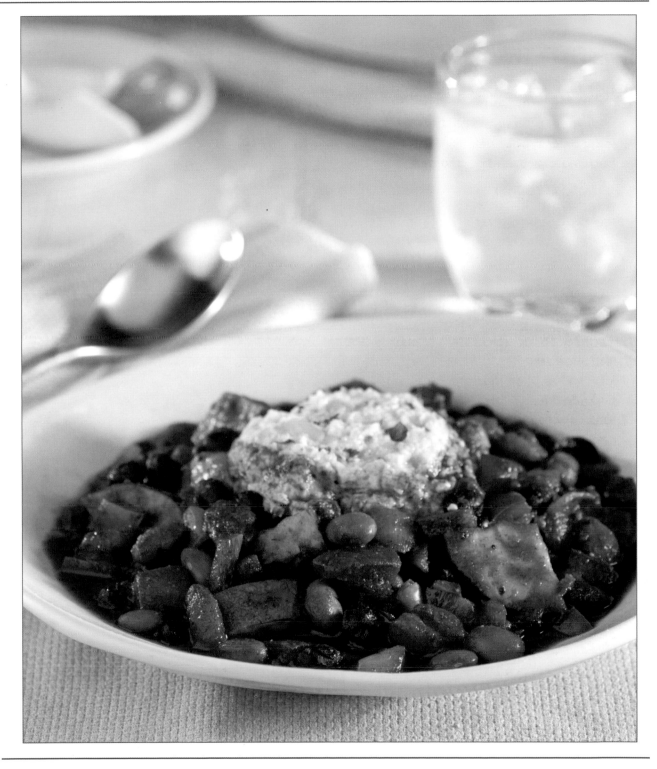

bean ragoût with cilantro-cornmeal dumplings, continued

3. Meanwhile, prepare dumplings. Combine flour blend, cornmeal, baking powder, xanthan gum and remaining ½ teaspoon salt in medium bowl; cut in shortening with pastry blender or two knives until mixture resembles coarse crumbs.

4. Stir in cheese and cilantro. Pour milk into flour mixture; stir just until dry ingredients are moistened.

5. Drop dough on top of simmering ragoût in 6 mounds. Cook, uncovered, 5 minutes. Cover; cook 5 to 10 minutes more or until wooden toothpick inserted into dumplings comes out clean.

Makes 6 servings

roasted almond tilapia dairy-free

   2 tilapia or Boston scrod fillets (6 ounces each)
¼ teaspoon salt
   1 tablespoon Dijon mustard
¼ cup rice flour
   2 tablespoons chopped almonds
      Paprika (optional)
      Lemon wedges

1. Preheat oven to 450°F. Place fish on small baking sheet; season with salt. Spread mustard over fish. Combine rice flour and almonds in small bowl; sprinkle over fish and press lightly. Sprinkle with paprika, if desired.

2. Bake 8 to 10 minutes or until fish is opaque in center and begins to flake when tested with fork. Serve with lemon wedges, if desired.

Makes 2 servings

spicy pork chop casserole

2 tablespoons olive oil, divided

2 cups frozen corn

2 cups frozen diced hash brown potatoes

1 can (about 14 ounces) diced tomatoes with basil, garlic and oregano, drained

2 teaspoons chili powder

1 teaspoon dried oregano

½ teaspoon ground cumin

⅛ teaspoon red pepper flakes

4 boneless pork loin chops (about 3 ounces each), cut about ¾ inch thick

¼ teaspoon black pepper

1. Preheat oven to 375°F. Coat 8-inch square baking dish or 2-quart casserole with cooking spray.

2. Heat 1 tablespoon olive oil in large nonstick skillet. Add corn; cook and stir over medium-high heat 5 minutes or until corn begins to brown. Add potatoes; cook and stir 5 minutes or until potatoes begin to brown. Stir in tomatoes, chili powder, oregano, cumin and red pepper flakes. Transfer to prepared baking dish.

3. Heat remaining 1 tablespoon oil over medium-high heat. Add pork; cook until browned on one side. Place browned side up on top of corn mixture in baking dish. Sprinkle with black pepper.

4. Bake 20 minutes or until pork is barely pink in center. Let stand 5 minutes before serving. *Makes 4 servings*

rosemary-garlic scallops with polenta

dairy-free

- 1 tablespoon olive oil
- 1 medium red bell pepper, sliced
- 1/3 cup chopped red onion
- 3 cloves garlic, minced
- 8 ounces bay scallops
- 2 teaspoons chopped fresh rosemary *or* 3/4 teaspoon dried rosemary
- 1/4 teaspoon black pepper
- 1 1/4 cups reduced-sodium chicken broth
- 1/2 cup cornmeal
- 1/4 teaspoon salt

1. Heat oil in large nonstick skillet over medium heat. Add bell pepper, onion and garlic; cook and stir 5 minutes. Add scallops, rosemary and black pepper; cook 3 to 5 minutes or until scallops are opaque, stirring occasionally.

2. Meanwhile, combine broth, cornmeal and salt in small saucepan. Bring to a boil over high heat. Reduce heat to low; simmer 5 minutes or until polenta is very thick, stirring frequently. Transfer to serving plates; top with scallop mixture.

Makes 2 servings

recipe notes

Bay scallops are tiny shellfish, about 1/2 inch in diameter. Their meat is sweeter than the larger sea scallop and also more expensive. Sea scallops average 1 1/2 inches in diameter. Scallops should be a creamy or light pink color. If they are stark white they have probably been soaked in water and a phosphate solution to make them absorb liquid and weigh more. To be certain you're not paying for water, choose scallops that are labelled as "dry packed."

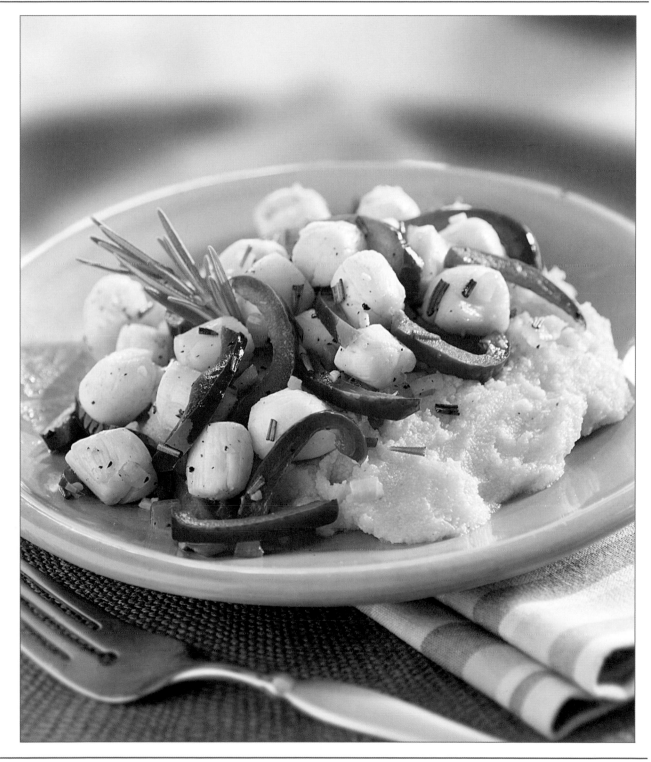

salmon-potato cakes with mustard tartar sauce

3 small unpeeled red potatoes (8 ounces), cut into halves
1 cup cooked flaked salmon
2 green onions, chopped
1 egg white
2 tablespoons chopped fresh parsley, divided
½ teaspoon Cajun seasoning
1 tablespoon olive oil
1 tablespoon mayonnaise
1 tablespoon plain yogurt or sour cream
2 teaspoons coarse grain mustard
1 tablespoon chopped dill pickle
1 teaspoon lemon juice

1. Place potatoes in small saucepan and cover with water. Bring to a boil; reduce heat and simmer about 15 minutes or until tender. Drain; mash with fork.

2. Combine potatoes, salmon, green onions, egg white, 1 tablespoon parsley and seasoning in medium bowl.

3. Heat oil in medium nonstick skillet over medium heat. Gently shape salmon mixture into 2 patties. Place in skillet; flatten slightly. Cook 7 minutes or until browned, turning once.

4. Meanwhile, combine mayonnaise, yogurt, mustard, pickle, lemon juice and remaining 1 tablespoon parsley in small bowl. Serve with cakes. *Makes 2 servings*

dairy-free variation

Serve salmon cakes with salsa or fruit chutney instead of mustard tartar sauce. Or prepare tartar sauce with dairy-free mayonnaise and soy or other dairy-free yogurt.

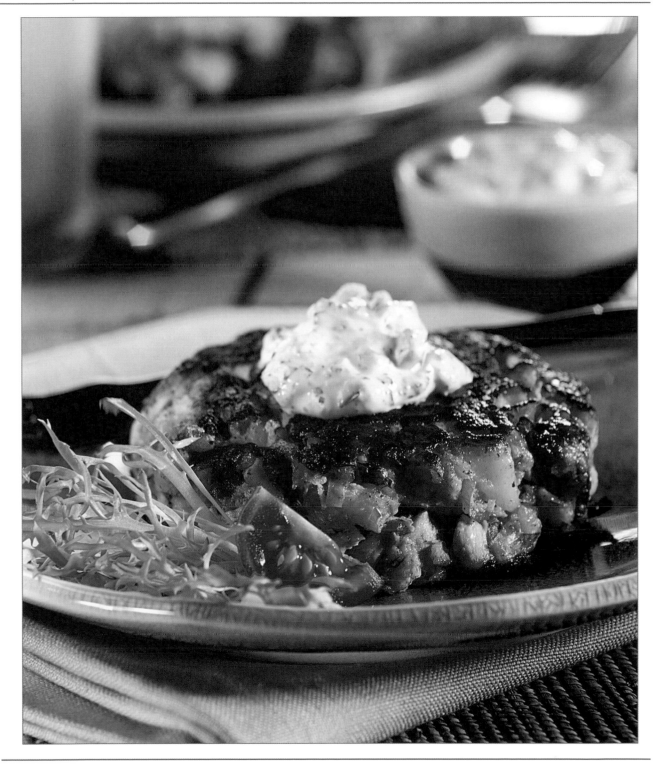

shepherd's pie

1 pound potatoes, peeled and quartered
2 to 3 tablespoons chicken broth
3 tablespoons grated Parmesan cheese
1 pound ground beef
½ cup chopped onion
2 teaspoons Italian seasoning
¼ teaspoon fennel seeds, crushed (optional)
⅛ teaspoon ground red pepper
2 cups sliced yellow summer squash
1 can (about 14 ounces) chunky pasta-style tomatoes, drained
1 cup corn
⅓ cup tomato paste

1. Preheat oven to 375°F. Combine potatoes and enough water to cover in medium saucepan. Bring to a boil. Boil, uncovered, 20 to 25 minutes or until tender; drain. Mash potatoes, adding enough broth to reach desired consistency. Stir in Parmesan cheese.

2. Meanwhile, brown beef and onion in large skillet over medium-high heat 6 to 8 minutes, stirring to break up meat. Drain fat. Stir in Italian seasoning, fennel seeds, if desired, and red pepper. Add squash, tomatoes, corn and tomato paste; mix well. Spoon into 2-quart casserole. Pipe or spoon potatoes over top.

3. Bake 20 to 25 minutes or until bubbly. Let stand 10 minutes before serving. *Makes 6 servings*

dairy-free variation

Omit Parmesan cheese or replace it with dairy-free cheese alternative.

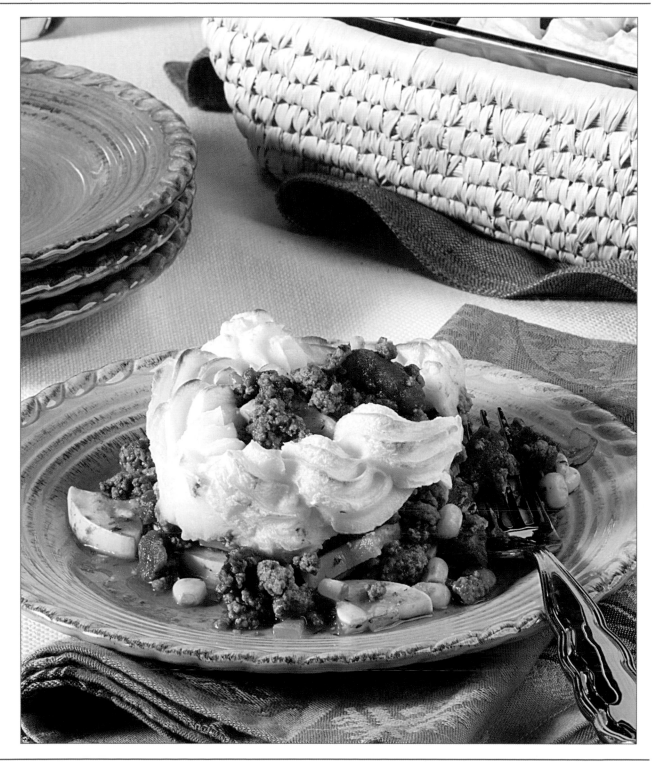

southwestern meat loaf

- **1 pound ground beef**
- **½ cup finely chopped onion**
- **½ cup cornmeal**
- **¼ cup chopped fresh cilantro leaves**
- **1 can (4 ounces) chopped mild green chiles, drained**
- **1 egg**
- **1½ teaspoons ground cumin**
- **¼ teaspoon salt**
- **¼ teaspoon black pepper**
- **1 can (8 ounces) tomato sauce, divided**
- **2 tablespoons ketchup**

1. Preheat oven to 350°F. Spray 13×9-inch baking pan with nonstick cooking spray.

2. Combine beef, onion, cornmeal, cilantro, chiles, egg, cumin, salt, pepper and half of tomato sauce in large bowl; mix well. Combine remaining tomato sauce and ketchup in small bowl.

3. Shape meat mixture into 6×9-inch oval in prepared baking pan. Top with tomato sauce mixture. Bake 55 minutes or until cooked through (160°F).

4. Let stand 5 minutes before slicing.

Makes 4 servings

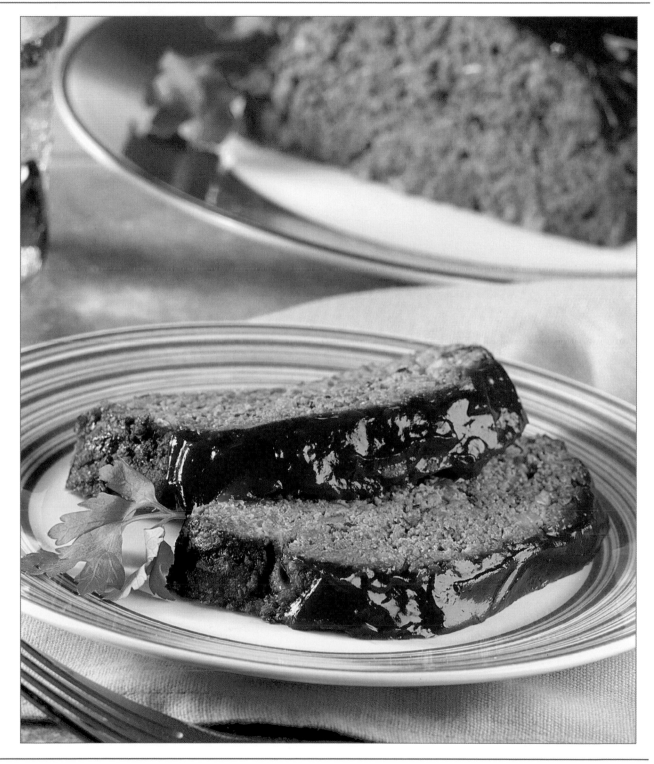

cheesy shrimp on grits

1 cup finely chopped green bell pepper

1 cup finely chopped red bell pepper

½ cup thinly sliced celery

1 cup chopped green onions, divided

4 tablespoons (½ stick) butter, cubed

1¼ teaspoons seafood seasoning

2 bay leaves

¼ teaspoon ground red pepper

1 pound uncooked shrimp, peeled and deveined

1⅓ cups quick-cooking corn grits

2 cups (8 ounces) shredded sharp Cheddar cheese

¼ cup whipping cream or half-and-half

slow cooker directions

1. Coat slow cooker with nonstick cooking spray. Add bell peppers, celery, ½ cup green onions, butter, seafood seasoning, bay leaves and ground red pepper. Cover; cook on LOW 4 hours or on HIGH 2 hours.

2. *Turn slow cooker to HIGH.* Add shrimp. Cover; cook 15 minutes. Meanwhile, prepare grits according to package directions.

3. Remove and discard bay leaves. Stir cheese, cream and remaining ½ cup green onions into slow cooker. Cook, uncovered, 5 minutes or until cheese melts. Serve over grits.

Makes 6 servings

gluten-free info

Grits, polenta and cornmeal are all ground corn. Although they can usually be used interchangeably, it's helpful to understand the terms. Grits are often labeled hominy grits and they are ground from dried corn that has been treated with slaked lime. This is the same process that gives corn tortillas their distinctive flavor. Cornmeal is ground dried corn and is available in a range of grinds. Whole grain cornmeal, which is usually stone ground, is more nutritious and flavorful than ordinary cornmeal, but also spoils much more quickly. Polenta is the name of an Italian dish made from cornmeal, which is eaten hot, or cooled, sliced and fried. In the U.S. we would call it cornmeal mush!

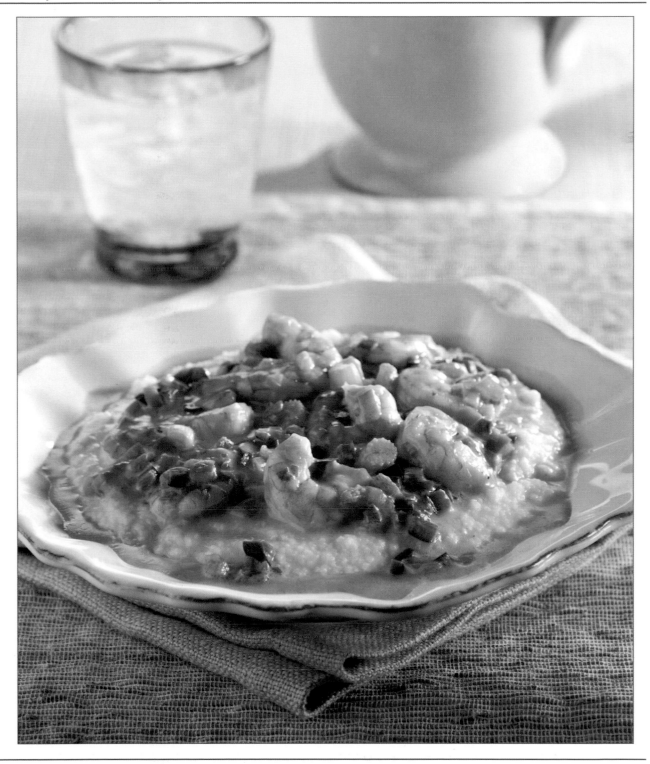

quinoa with roasted vegetables

 dairy-free

Nonstick cooking spray

2 medium sweet potatoes, cut into ½-inch-thick slices

1 medium eggplant, peeled and cut into ½-inch cubes

1 medium tomato, cut into wedges

1 large green bell pepper, sliced

1 small onion, cut into wedges

½ teaspoon salt

¼ teaspoon black pepper

¼ teaspoon ground red pepper

1 cup uncooked quinoa

2 cloves garlic, minced

½ teaspoon dried thyme

¼ teaspoon dried marjoram

2 cups water or vegetable broth

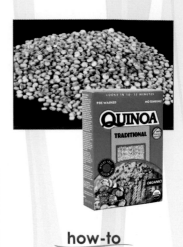

1. Preheat oven to 450°F. Line large jelly-roll pan with foil; spray with cooking spray.

2. Arrange sweet potatoes, eggplant, tomato, bell pepper and onion on prepared pan; spray lightly with cooking spray. Sprinkle with salt, black pepper and ground red pepper; toss to coat. Bake 20 to 30 minutes or until vegetables are browned and tender.

3. Meanwhile, place quinoa in fine-mesh strainer; rinse well under cold running water. Spray medium saucepan with cooking spray; heat over medium heat. Add garlic, thyme and marjoram; cook and stir 1 to 2 minutes. Add quinoa; cook and stir 2 to 3 minutes. Stir in water; bring to a boil over high heat. Reduce heat to low. Simmer, covered, 15 to 20 minutes or until water is absorbed. Transfer quinoa to large bowl; gently stir in vegetables.

Makes 6 servings

how-to

Quinoa is usually rinsed before using. The seeds are naturally coated with a substance called saponin, which protects quinoa from insects while it's growing. The grain is almost always rinsed once before packaging to remove the bitter saponin, but it doesn't hurt to rinse quinoa again before using it. Place it in a fine-mesh strainer and swish the grains around under cold running water. If the water looks cloudy or soapy, that's the saponin.

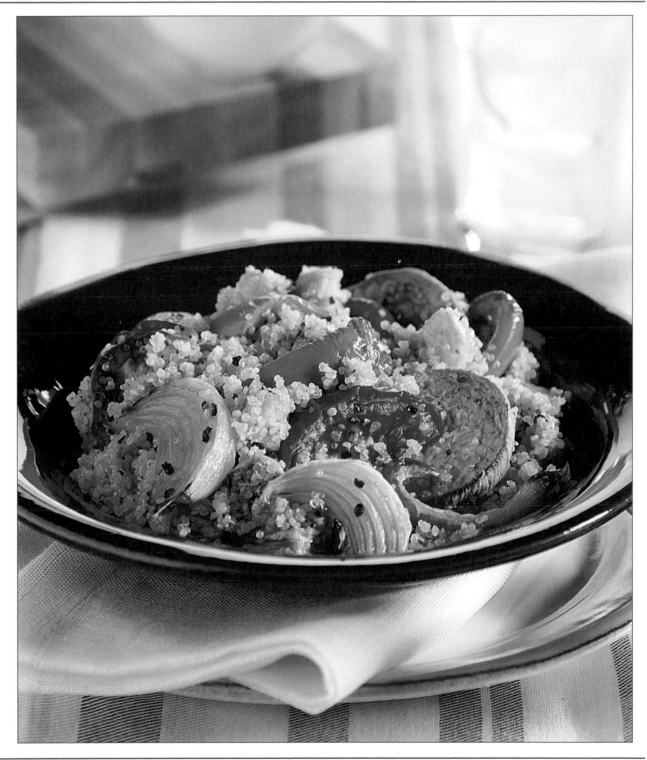

cajun chicken & rice

dairy-free

4 chicken drumsticks, skin removed
4 chicken thighs, skin removed
2 teaspoons Cajun seasoning
¾ teaspoon salt
2 tablespoons vegetable oil
1 can (about 14 ounces) chicken broth
1 cup uncooked rice
1 medium green bell pepper, coarsely chopped
1 medium red bell pepper, coarsely chopped
½ cup finely chopped green onions
2 cloves garlic, minced
½ teaspoon dried thyme
¼ teaspoon ground turmeric

1. Preheat oven to 350°F. Lightly coat 13×9-inch baking dish with nonstick cooking spray.

2. Sprinkle both sides of chicken with Cajun seasoning and salt. Heat oil in large skillet over medium-high heat. Add chicken; cook 8 to 10 minutes or until browned on all sides. Remove from skillet.

3. Add broth to skillet; bring to a boil, scraping brown bits from bottom of skillet. Stir in rice, bell peppers, green onions, garlic, thyme and turmeric. Pour into prepared baking dish. Place chicken on top. Cover tightly with foil. Bake 1 hour or until chicken is cooked through (165°F). *Makes 6 servings*

variation

For a one-dish meal, use an ovenproof skillet. Place browned chicken on mixture in skillet, cover and bake as directed.

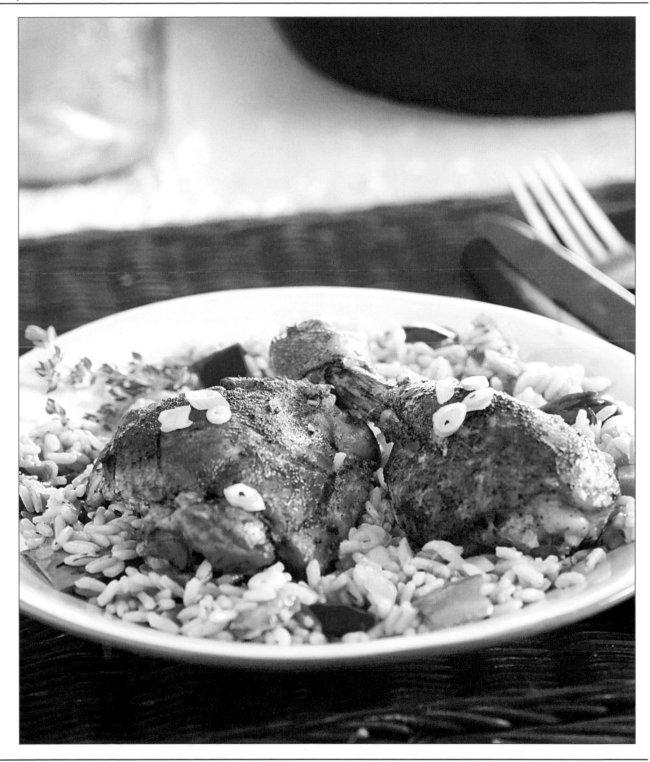

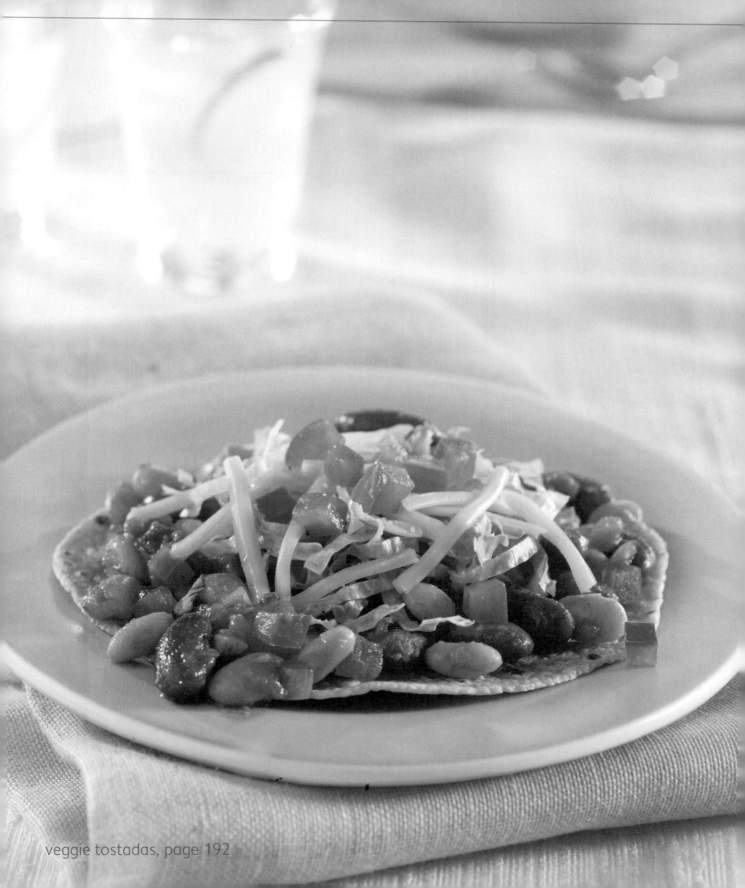

veggie tostadas, page 192

ethnic adventures

Take a tasty trip around the world to sample cuisines that don't depend on gluten. There are luscious Asian rice noodle dishes, creamy Italian risottos, spicy Mexican tamales and so much more. These recipes make gluten-free eating a delightful adventure in flavor.

vietnamese beef soup

 dairy-free

¾ **pound boneless beef top sirloin or top round steak**

6 **cups beef broth**

3 **cups water**

2 **tablespoons gluten-free soy sauce**

2 **tablespoons minced fresh ginger**

1 **cinnamon stick (3 inches long)**

4 **ounces rice noodles (see sidebar)**

½ **cup thinly sliced or julienned carrots**

2 **cups fresh bean sprouts**

1 **small red onion, halved and thinly sliced**

½ **cup chopped fresh cilantro**

½ **cup chopped fresh basil**

2 **jalapeño peppers,* minced**

*Jalapeño peppers can sting and irritate the skin, so wear rubber gloves when handling peppers and do not touch your eyes.

1. Freeze beef 45 minutes or until firm.

2. Combine broth, water, soy sauce, ginger and cinnamon stick in large saucepan; bring to a boil over high heat. Reduce heat to low; simmer, covered, 20 to 30 minutes. Remove cinnamon stick; discard.

3. Meanwhile, place rice noodles in large bowl. Cover with hot water; let stand 15 to 20 minutes or until softened. Drain

4. Slice beef lengthwise in half, then crosswise into very thin strips. Add noodles and carrots to simmering broth; cook 2 to 3 minutes or until carrots are tender. Add beef and bean sprouts; cook 1 minute or until beef is no longer pink.

5. Remove from heat; stir in red onion, cilantro, basil and jalapeño peppers.

Makes 6 servings

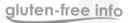

gluten-free info

Rice noodles are semi-translucent dried noodles that come in many sizes and have many names, including rice stick noodles, rice-flour noodles and pho noodles. (This soup is called "pho" in Vietnamese.) Widths range from string thin (usually called rice vermicelli) to 1 inch wide. All rice noodles must be soaked to soften before using and all may be used interchangeably.

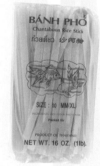

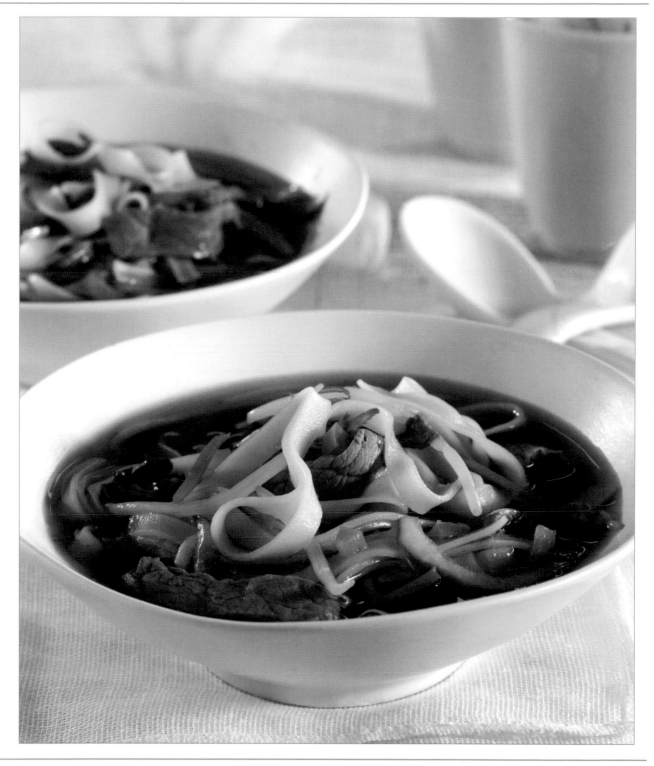

tamales

1 package dried corn husks

4 ounces quesadilla cheese or mozzarella cheese

1 can (about 7 ounces) pickled jalapeños, drained

1 can (about 15 ounces) yellow corn, drained, liquid reserved

1 to 1½ cups cornmeal

2 tablespoons softened butter

1 teaspoon salt

Salsa, pico de gallo or guacamole

1. Soak corn husks in hot water 1 hour or until softened.

2. Cut cheese into 4-inch long strips. Cut jalapeños into strips. Tear narrow strips of corn husk to use as ties for tamales.*

3. Place corn and 2 tablespoons reserved corn liquid in food processor. Pulse until paste forms. Add 1 cup cornmeal, butter and salt. Pulse 1 minute or until dough forms. Add more cornmeal gradually until dough is soft and moist, but not sticky. Transfer dough to work surface and keep covered to prevent drying out.

4. Pat corn husk dry and place on work surface. Place 2 tablespoons of cornmeal mixture in center of husk. Pat dough into a rectangle about 4×2 inches. Arrange 1 strip of cheese and 1 strip of jalapeño in center of dough.

5. Lift sides of husk to enclose filling in dough and wrap gently around tamale. Fold bottom of husk over tamale; tie closed with strip of husk. Tie top closed or leave open. Transfer tamales to steamer basket.

6. Fill large saucepan with water to a depth that will not touch bottom of steamer basket. Bring to a boil. Place steamer basket over water. Cover; steam 45 minutes to 1 hour or until tamale no longer sticks to corn husk, adding additional water to saucepan as needed.

7. Serve tamales with salsa. Tamales may also be refrigerated or frozen and reheated in steamer or microwave.

Makes 8 tamales

Or secure tamales with kitchen twine.

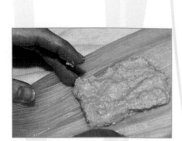

Pat dough into rectangle.

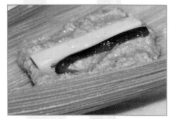

Arrange cheese and jalapeños in center.

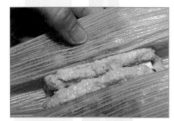

Fold corn husk around filling.

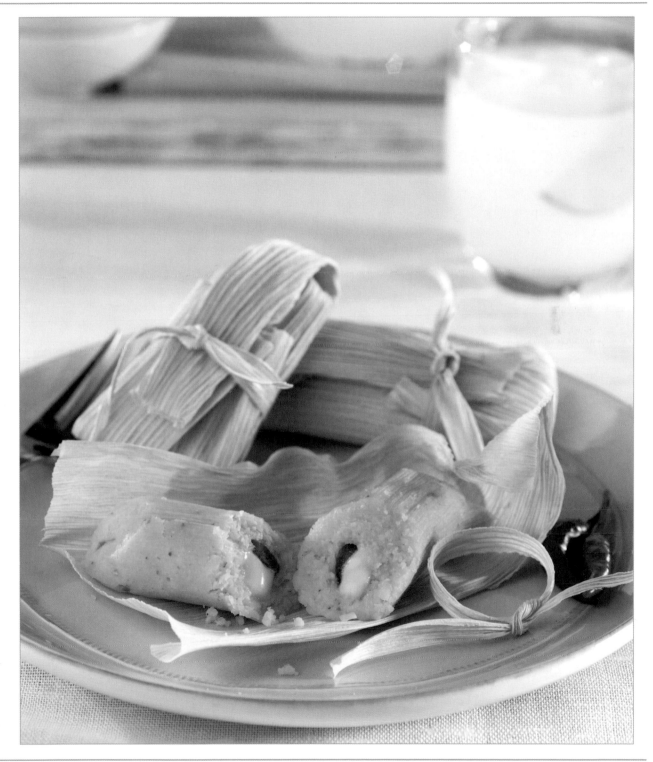

mexican tortilla stack-ups

1 tablespoon vegetable oil

½ cup chopped onion

1 can (about 15 ounces) black beans, rinsed and drained

1 can (14½ ounces) Mexican- or Italian-style diced tomatoes

1 cup frozen corn

1 package (1¼ ounces) gluten-free taco seasoning mix

6 (6-inch) corn tortillas

2 cups (8 ounces) taco-flavored shredded Cheddar cheese

1 cup water

Sliced black olives (optional)

1. Preheat oven to 350°F. Spray 13×9-inch baking dish with nonstick cooking spray.

2. Heat oil in large skillet over medium-high heat. Add onion; cook and stir 3 minutes or until tender. Add beans, tomatoes, corn and taco seasoning mix. Bring to a boil over high heat. Reduce heat to low; simmer 5 minutes.

3. Place 2 tortillas side by side in prepared dish. Top each tortilla with about ½ cup bean mixture. Sprinkle evenly with one third of cheese. Repeat layers twice, creating 2 tortilla stacks each 3 tortillas high. Pour water along sides of tortillas.

4. Cover tightly with foil and bake 30 to 35 minutes or until heated through. Cut into wedges to serve. Top with black olives.

Makes 6 servings

gluten-free info

Corn tortillas are the everyday bread of Mexico and a must for any gluten-free kitchen. Tortillas can be wrapped, stacked, deep-fried or used to replace bread. If you live near a Latin American market, you'll be able to sample different brands of fresh corn tortillas.

A word of warning, however—a few brands of corn tortillas may contain wheat flour, so double check. It's another example of the growing trend to add gluten to all sorts of products.

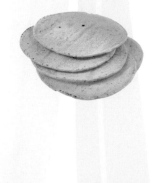

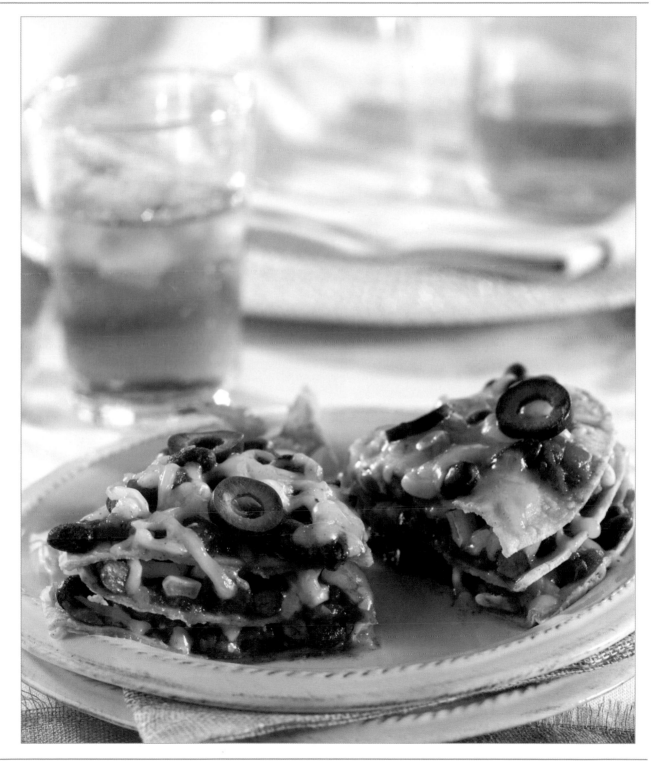

polenta with pasta sauce & vegetables

1 can (about 14 ounces) vegetable broth

1½ cups water

1 cup yellow cornmeal

2 teaspoons olive oil

12 ounces assorted cut-up vegetables, such as broccoli florets, bell peppers, red onions, zucchini squash and thin carrot strips

2 teaspoons minced garlic

2 cups prepared tomato-basil pasta sauce

½ cup grated Asiago cheese

¼ cup chopped fresh basil (optional)

1. To prepare polenta, whisk together broth, water and cornmeal in large microwavable bowl. Cover with waxed paper; microwave on HIGH 5 minutes. Whisk well and microwave on HIGH 4 to 5 minutes more or until polenta is very thick. Whisk again; cover and keep warm.

2. Meanwhile, heat oil in large deep nonstick skillet over medium heat. Add vegetables and garlic; cook and stir 5 minutes. Add pasta sauce. Reduce heat; cover and simmer 5 to 8 minutes or until vegetables are tender.

3. Spoon polenta onto serving plates; top with pasta sauce mixture. Sprinkle with cheese and basil.   *Makes 4 servings*

dairy-free variation

Omit Asiago cheese or replace it with a dairy-free cheese alternative.

gluten-free info

Polenta is simply the Italian word for cornmeal mush. The texture and flavor can be varied by using different sorts of cornmeal, changing the liquid or adding less of it. If you prefer, you could also make this polenta in a saucepan. Bring the liquid to a boil and gradually add the cornmeal in a steady stream, whisking constantly. Reduce the heat to medium and cook, stirring occasionally, until the polenta is thickened.

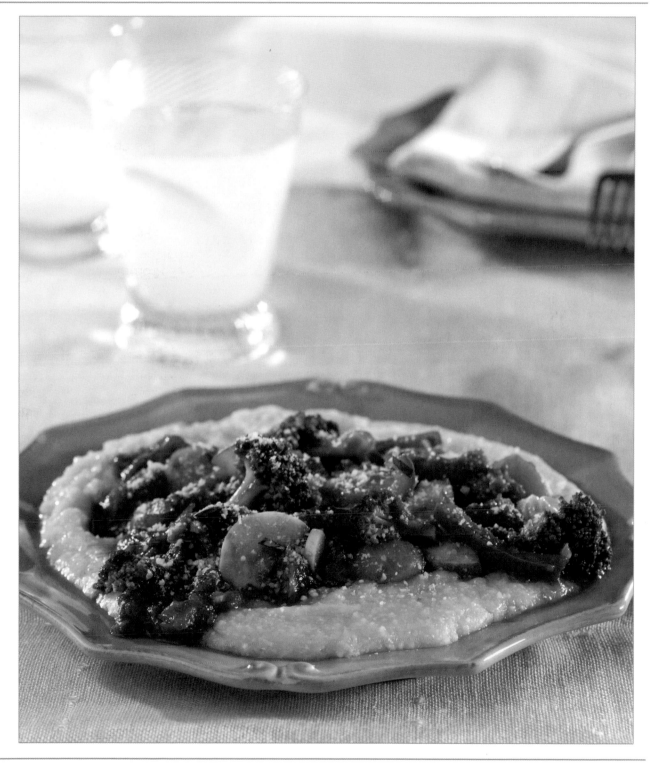

veggie tostadas

[pictured on page 182]

- **1 tablespoon olive oil**
- **1 cup chopped onion**
- **1 cup chopped celery**
- **2 cloves garlic, chopped**
- **1 can (about 15 ounces) red kidney beans, rinsed and drained**
- **1 can (about 15 ounces) Great Northern beans, rinsed and drained**
- **1 can (14½ ounces) salsa-style diced tomatoes**
- **2 teaspoons mild chili powder**
- **1 teaspoon ground cumin**
- **6 (6-inch) corn tortillas**
- **Toppings: Chopped fresh cilantro, shredded lettuce, chopped seeded fresh tomatoes, shredded Cheddar cheese and sour cream**

1. Heat oil in large skillet over medium heat. Add onion, celery and garlic. Cook and stir 8 minutes or until softened. Stir in beans, tomatoes, chili powder and cumin. Reduce heat to medium-low. Simmer 30 minutes, stirring occasionally, until thickened.

2. Meanwhile, preheat oven to 400°F. Place tortillas in single layer directly on oven rack. Bake 10 to 12 minutes or until crisp. Place one tortilla on each plate. Spoon bean mixture evenly over each tortilla. Top with cilantro, lettuce, tomatoes, Cheddar cheese and sour cream, if desired.

Makes 6 servings

dairy-free variation

Omit cheese and sour cream or replace with dairy-free alternatives.

chicken saltimbocca

 dairy-free

¼ **cup coarsely chopped fresh basil**

2 **tablespoons minced fresh chives**

2 **teaspoons extra virgin olive oil**

1 **clove garlic, minced**

½ **teaspoon dried oregano**

½ **teaspoon dried sage**

4 **boneless skinless chicken breasts (about 4 ounces each)**

2 **slices (1 ounce each) smoked ham, cut in half**

  Nonstick cooking spray

½ **cup chicken broth**

1 **cup pasta sauce**

2 **cups hot cooked spaghetti squash (see sidebar)**

1. Combine basil, chives, oil, garlic, oregano and sage in small bowl. Pound chicken between waxed paper to ½- to ¾-inch thickness with flat side of meat mallet or rolling pin. Spread herb mixture evenly over chicken. Place 1 ham slice over herb mixture; roll up to enclose filling. Secure with toothpicks.

2. Spray medium nonstick skillet with cooking spray; heat over medium-high heat. Cook chicken, seam side up, 2 to 3 minutes or until browned. Turn; cook 2 to 3 minutes or until browned. Add broth; reduce heat to medium-low. Cover and simmer 20 minutes or until cooked through.

3. Remove chicken to cutting board, leaving liquid in skillet. Let chicken stand 5 minutes. Add pasta sauce to same skillet; cook over medium-low heat 2 to 3 minutes or until heated through, stirring occasionally.

4. Remove toothpicks from chicken and cut crosswise into slices. Serve chicken with squash. Top with sauce. *Makes 4 servings*

how-to

To cook spaghetti squash, cut the squash in half lengthwise. Remove and discard the seeds. Place, cut side down, in a microwavable baking dish. Add ½ cup water. Cover; cook on HIGH 10 to 15 minutes or until soft. Let cool 15 minutes. Scrape out squash "strands" with a fork. Makes about 4 cups cooked squash.

vietnamese summer rolls

dairy-free

Vietnamese Dipping Sauce (recipe follows)
8 ounces medium raw shrimp, peeled and deveined
3½ ounces thin rice noodles (rice vermicelli)
12 rice paper wrappers,* about 6½ inches in diameter
36 whole fresh cilantro leaves
4 ounces roast pork or beef, sliced ⅛ inch thick
1 tablespoon chopped peanuts
Lime peel (optional)

Available at specialty stores or Asian markets. Rice paper is a thin, edible wrapper used in Southeast Asian cooking.

1. Prepare Vietnamese Dipping Sauce; set aside.

2. Bring large saucepan of water to a boil over high heat. Add shrimp; simmer 1 to 2 minutes or until shrimp turn pink and opaque. Remove shrimp with slotted spoon to small bowl. Slice shrimp in half lengthwise when cool enough to handle.

3. Meanwhile, place rice noodles in medium bowl; cover with hot water. Soak 15 minutes or until softened. Drain; cut into 3-inch pieces.

4. Soften rice paper wrapper in large bowl of warm water 30 to 40 seconds or until pliable. Drain on paper towel and transfer to work surface. Arrange 3 cilantro leaves in center of wrapper. Layer with two shrimp halves, pork and rice noodles.

5. Fold bottom of wrapper over filling; fold in each side and roll up. Repeat with remaining wrappers.

6. Sprinkle Summer Rolls with peanuts. Serve with Vietnamese Dipping Sauce. Garnish with lime peel.   *Makes 12 summer rolls*

vietnamese dipping sauce: Combine ½ cup water, ¼ cup gluten-free fish sauce, 2 tablespoons lime juice, 1 tablespoon sugar, 1 clove garlic, minced, and ¼ teaspoon chili oil in small bowl.

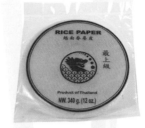
Rice paper wrappers are available at Asian markets.

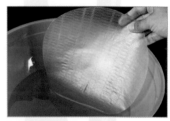
Soften rice paper wrappers in warm water.

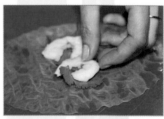
Arrange ingredients in center.

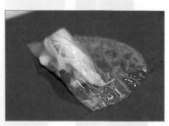
Roll up wrapper.

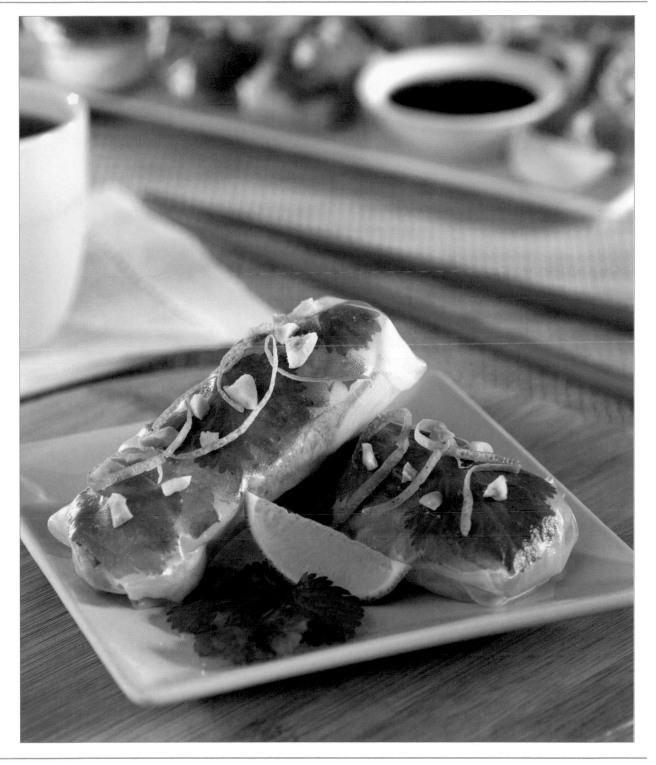

south american chicken & quinoa

dairy-free

1 teaspoon ground turmeric

1 teaspoon dried thyme

¾ teaspoon salt, divided

1 pound boneless skinless chicken breasts, cut into 1-inch pieces

2 tablespoons olive oil, divided

1 red bell pepper, chopped

1 medium onion, chopped

1 cup uncooked quinoa

1 cup chicken broth

1 cup unsweetened coconut milk

1 teaspoon curry powder

¼ teaspoon ground ginger

1. Combine turmeric, thyme and ¼ teaspoon salt in shallow dish. Dip chicken pieces into spice mixture, coating all sides; set aside.

2. Heat 1 tablespoon oil in large skillet over medium-high heat. Add bell pepper and onion. Cook and stir 2 minutes or until vegetables are crisp-tender. Remove from skillet with slotted spoon; set aside.

3. Add remaining 1 tablespoon oil and chicken to skillet. Cook and stir 5 minutes or until browned and cooked through.

4. Rinse quinoa in fine-mesh strainer under cold running water; drain well.

5. Combine quinoa, chicken broth, coconut milk, curry powder, ginger and remaining ½ teaspoon salt in large saucepan. Bring to a boil over high heat. Reduce heat to low; simmer, covered, 10 minutes.

6. Stir in chicken and pepper mixture; cook 5 minutes or until liquid is absorbed.   *Makes 4 servings*

gluten-free info

Quinoa is usually rinsed before using. The seeds are naturally coated with a substance called saponin, which protects quinoa from insects while it's growing. The grain is almost always rinsed once before packaging to remove the bitter saponin, but it doesn't hurt to rinse quinoa again before using it. Place it in a fine-mesh strainer and swish the grains around under cold running water. If the water looks cloudy or soapy, that's the saponin.

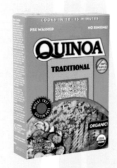

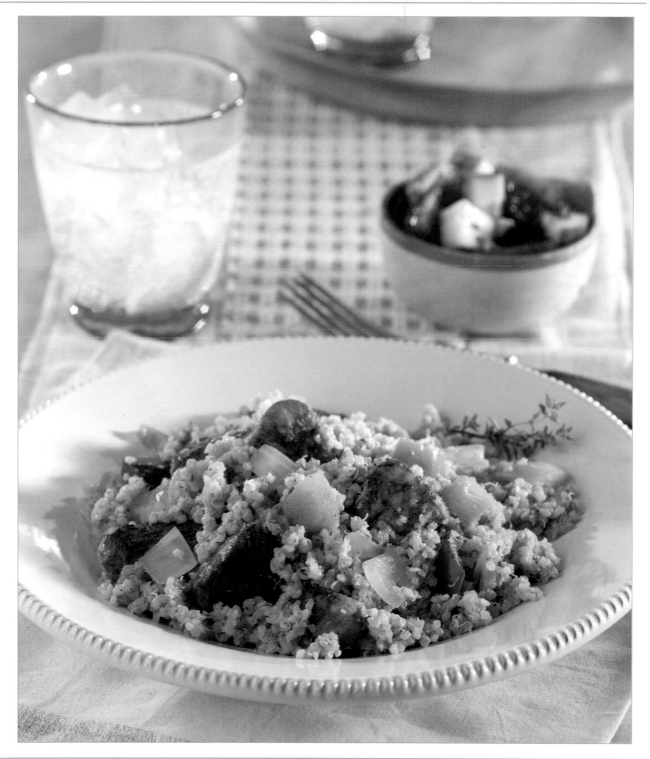

fiesta beef enchiladas

6 ounces ground beef

¼ cup sliced green onions

1 teaspoon minced garlic

1 cup (4 ounces) shredded Mexican cheese blend or Cheddar cheese, divided

1 cup chopped tomato, divided

½ cup corn

⅓ cup cooked rice

½ cup black beans

¼ cup salsa or picante sauce

6 (6-inch) corn tortillas

½ cup gluten-free enchilada sauce

Sliced lettuce

dairy-free variation

Replace cheese with a dairy-free cheese alternative.

1. Preheat oven to 375°F. Spray two 20×12-inch sheets of heavy duty foil with nonstick cooking spray.

2. Brown ground beef in large nonstick skillet over medium-heat, stirring to separate meat. Drain fat. Add green onions and garlic; cook and stir 2 minutes.

3. Combine meat mixture, ¾ cup cheese, ½ cup tomato, corn, rice, beans and salsa; mix well. Spoon mixture down center of tortillas. Roll up; place 3 enchiladas, seam side down, on each foil sheet. Top with enchilada sauce.

4. Seal packets, leaving head space for heat circulation. Place on baking sheet. Bake 15 minutes.

5. Remove from oven; open packets. Sprinkle with remaining ¼ cup cheese. Reseal packets. Bake 10 minutes or until cheese melts. Serve with lettuce and remaining ½ cup tomato.

Makes 2 servings

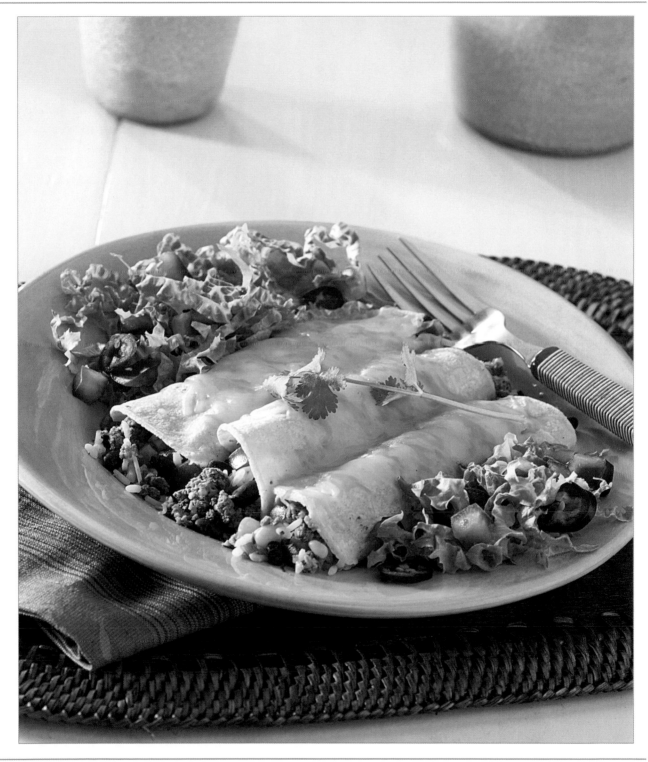

sizzling rice flour crêpes

dairy-free

crêpes

    1 cup rice flour
    ½ teaspoon salt
    ½ teaspoon sugar
    ½ teaspoon turmeric
    1 cup unsweetened coconut milk
    ½ to ¾ cup water
    ½ cup vegetable oil

dipping sauce

    ⅔ cup water
    ¼ cup gluten-free fish sauce
    2 tablespoons sugar
       Juice of 1 lime
    1 clove garlic, minced
    1 serrano or other hot pepper, minced
    1 to 2 tablespoons shredded carrot

filling and garnishes

    1 bunch green onions, chopped
    1 cup chopped cooked chicken, small raw shrimp, peeled or
       cubed tofu
    2 cups bean sprouts
       Lettuce, fresh cilantro and fresh mint

1. Combine rice flour, salt, sugar and turmeric in medium bowl. Gradually whisk in coconut milk and ½ cup water until batter is thickness of heavy cream. Let batter rest at least 10 minutes. Add additional water as needed to thin batter.

2. For dipping sauce, combine ⅔ cup water, fish sauce, sugar and lime juice in small bowl. Stir until sugar dissolves. Stir in garlic and pepper; top with carrot. Set aside.

continued on page 202

Sizzling Crêpes (Banh Xeo, pronounced bahn SAY-oh) are a popular Vietnamese street snack. The word "Xeo" in Vietnamese mimics the sound the batter makes as it sizzles in the pan. The filling can be almost anything you wish. Try using leftover pork, beef, vegetables or whatever you have on hand. Part of the experience is choosing which fresh herbs to add to each portion of crêpe before wrapping it in a lettuce leaf and dipping it in sauce. Banh Xeo are a truly hands-on eating experience!

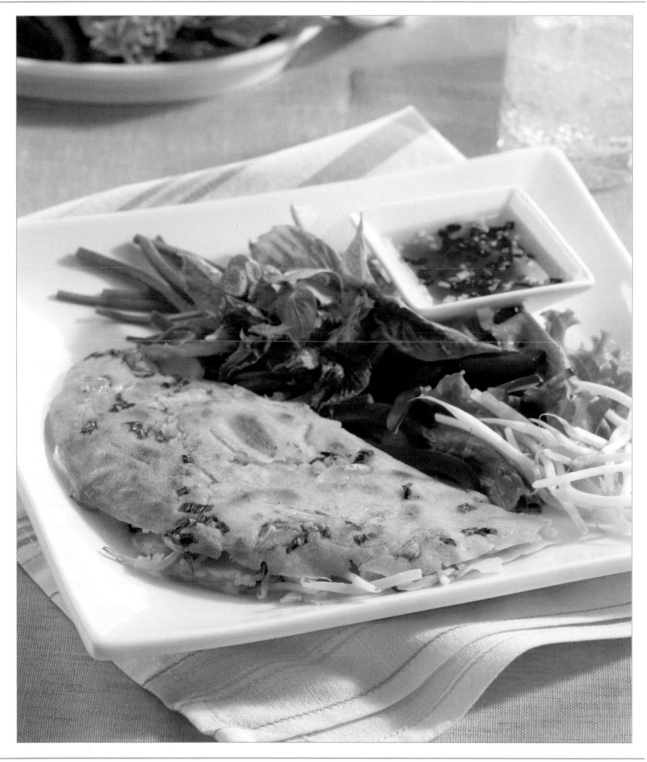

sizzling rice flour crêpes, continued

3. Heat 3 teaspoons oil in 9- or 10-inch nonstick skillet over medium heat. Add choice of ¼ cup filling to skillet: about 1 tablespoon green onion, plus 3 tablespoons chicken, shrimp, tofu or a combination. Cook and stir 2 to 4 minutes or until onions are softened and shrimp is pink and opaque. Pour about ½ cup batter over filling mixture. Immediately swirl to coat bottom of pan with batter; allow some batter to go up side of pan.

4. In 30 seconds or when sizzling sound stops, add bean sprouts to one side of crêpe. Cover pan and cook 3 minutes or until sprouts wilt and center of crêpe appears cooked. Edges should be browned and crisp.

5. Fold crêpe in half with spatula and transfer to plate. Repeat with remaining oil, batter and fillings.

6. Serve crêpes with lettuce, herbs and dipping sauce. Traditionally, crêpes are eaten by wrapping bite-size portions in lettuce with herbs and dipping each bite in sauce. *Makes 4 to 6 servings*

spinach & mushroom enchiladas

2 packages (10 ounces each) frozen chopped spinach, thawed and squeezed dry

1½ cups sliced mushrooms

1 can (about 15 ounces) pinto beans, rinsed and drained

3 teaspoons chili powder, divided

¼ teaspoon red pepper flakes

1 can (8 ounces) tomato sauce

2 tablespoons water

½ teaspoon hot pepper sauce

8 (8-inch) corn tortillas

1 cup (4 ounces) shredded Monterey Jack cheese

Toppings: shredded lettuce, chopped tomatoes, sour cream and chopped fresh cilantro (optional)

dairy-free variation

Replace cheese with a dairy-free cheese alternative.

1. Cook and stir spinach, mushrooms, beans, 2 teaspoons chili powder and red pepper flakes in large skillet over medium heat 5 minutes.

2. Combine tomato sauce, water, remaining 1 teaspoon chili powder and hot sauce in medium pan. Dip tortillas into tomato sauce mixture; stack tortillas on waxed paper.

3. Spoon filling into center of tortillas; roll up and place, seam side down, in 11×8-inch microwavable dish. Secure rolls with toothpicks, if necessary. Spread remaining tomato sauce mixture over enchiladas.

4. Cover with vented plastic wrap. Microwave on MEDIUM (50%) 10 minutes or until heated through. Sprinkle with cheese. Microwave on MEDIUM (50%) 3 minutes or until cheese is melted. Serve with lettuce, tomatoes, sour cream and cilantro, if desired.

Makes 4 servings

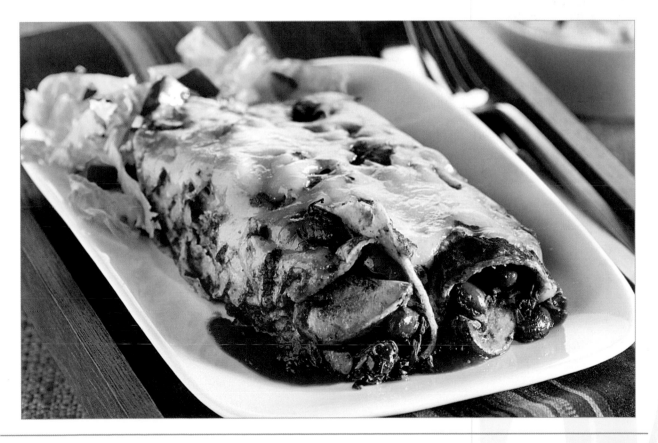

cheese soufflé

¼ **cup (½ stick) butter**
¼ **cup sweet rice flour (mochiko) (see sidebar)**
1½ **cups milk, warmed to room temperature**
¼ **teaspoon salt**
¼ **teaspoon ground red pepper**
⅛ **teaspoon black pepper**
6 **eggs, separated**
1 **cup (4 ounces) shredded Cheddar cheese**
Pinch cream of tartar (optional)

1. Preheat oven to 375°F. Grease four individual 2-cup soufflé dishes or one 2-quart soufflé dish.

2. Melt butter in large saucepan over medium-low heat. Add rice flour. Whisk 2 minutes or until mixture just begins to color. Whisk in milk. Add salt, red pepper and black pepper. Whisk until mixture comes to a boil and thickens. Remove from heat.

3. Stir in egg yolks, one at a time. Add cheese; stir until melted.

4. Meanwhile, place egg whites in clean large bowl with cream of tartar. Beat with electric mixer at high speed until egg whites form stiff peaks.

5. Fold egg whites into cheese mixture gently until almost combined. (Some streaks of white should remain.) Transfer mixture to prepared dish.

6. Bake about 20 minutes for individual soufflés or 30 to 40 minutes for larger soufflé or until puffed and browned. Wooden skewer inserted into center should come out moist, but clean. Serve immediately. *Makes 4 servings*

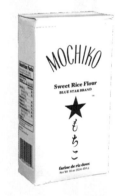

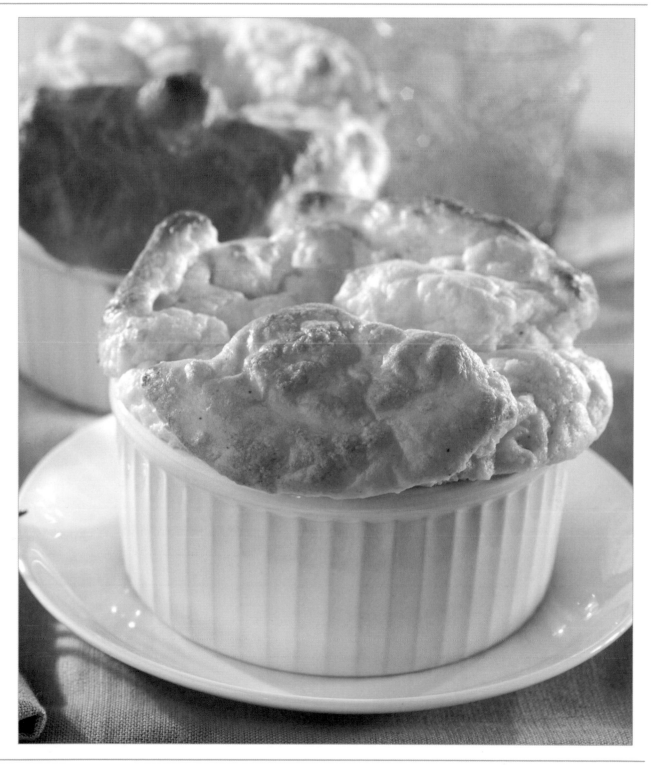

sukiyaki

dairy-free

1 package (3¾ ounces) cellophane noodles (bean threads)

½ cup beef broth

½ cup gluten-free teriyaki sauce

¼ cup sake, rice wine or dry sherry

1 tablespoon sugar

2 tablespoons vegetable oil

1 pound beef tenderloin or top sirloin steaks, cut crosswise into very thin strips

6 ounces fresh shiitake mushrooms, stemmed and sliced

8 ounces firm tofu, drained and cut into 1-inch cubes

6 green onions, cut into 2-inch pieces

½ pound fresh spinach, stems removed

1. Place noodles in bowl; cover with hot water. Let stand 15 minutes or until softened; drain. Cut into 4-inch pieces; set aside.

2. Combine broth, teriyaki sauce, sake and sugar in small bowl; mix well. Set aside.

3. Heat 1 tablespoon oil in wok or large skillet over high heat. Add half of beef; stir-fry 3 minutes or until browned. Remove to bowl. Repeat with remaining 1 tablespoon oil and beef.

4. Reduce heat to medium. Add mushrooms to wok; stir-fry 1 minute and move to side of wok. Add tofu; stir-fry 1 minute. Move to side of wok. Add green onions and broth mixture; bring to a boil. Move onions to side of wok.

5. Add noodles and spinach; stir gently. Add beef and juices. Stir ingredients together and heat through. *Makes 4 servings*

gluten-free info

Cellophane noodles are also called bean threads or glass noodles. Since they are made from mung bean flour, they are a good addition to the gluten-free pantry. Cellophane noodles are usually sold in tangled bunches and must be soaked before using.

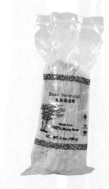

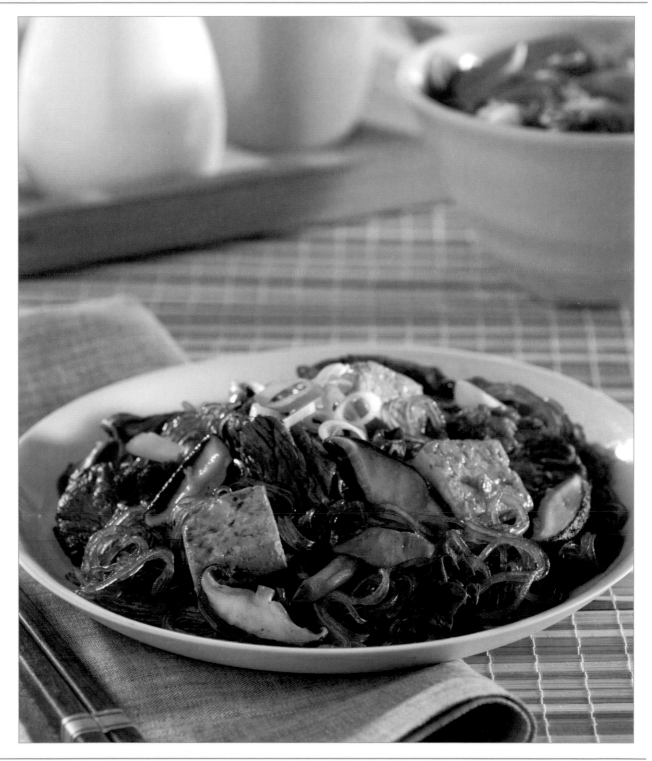

asparagus-parmesan risotto

  4 tablespoons unsalted butter, divided
⅓ cup finely chopped onion
  2 cups uncooked arborio rice
⅔ cup dry white wine
5½ cups vegetable broth
2½ cups fresh asparagus pieces (about 1 inch long)
⅔ cup frozen peas
  1 cup grated Parmesan cheese
    Salt and black pepper
    Shaved Parmesan cheese (optional)

1. Melt 3 tablespoons butter in large saucepan over medium heat. Add onion; cook and stir 2 to 3 minutes or until tender. Stir in rice; cook 2 minutes or until rice is coated with butter, stirring frequently. Add wine; cook, stirring occasionally, until most of wine is absorbed.

2. Bring broth to a simmer in medium saucepan over medium-high heat; reduce heat to low.

3. Add 1½ cups hot broth to rice mixture; cook and stir 6 to 7 minutes or until most of liquid is absorbed. (Mixture should simmer, but not boil.) Add 2 cups broth and asparagus; cook and stir 6 to 7 minutes or until most of liquid is absorbed. Add remaining 2 cups broth and peas; cook and stir 5 to 6 minutes or until most of liquid is absorbed and rice mixture is creamy.

4. Remove from heat; stir in remaining 1 tablespoon butter and Parmesan cheese until melted. Season to taste with salt and pepper. Garnish with shaved Parmesan.   *Makes 4 servings*

variations

asparagus-spinach risotto: Substitute 1 cup baby spinach leaves or chopped large spinach leaves for peas. Proceed as directed.

asparagus-chicken risotto: Add 2 cups chopped or shredded cooked chicken to risotto with the peas in step 3. Proceed as directed.

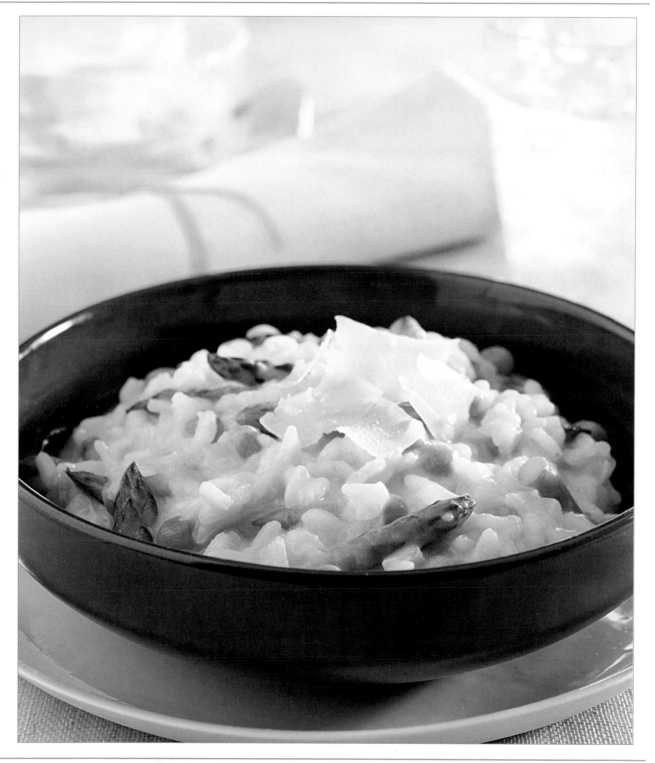

lemon-ginger chicken with puffed rice noodles

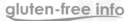
dairy-free

Vegetable oil for frying

4 ounces thin rice noodles, broken in half

3 boneless skinless chicken breasts, cut into bite-size pieces

1 stalk lemongrass, cut into 1-inch pieces

3 cloves garlic, minced

1 teaspoon finely chopped fresh ginger

¼ teaspoon ground red pepper

¼ teaspoon black pepper

¼ cup water

1 tablespoon cornstarch

2 tablespoons peanut oil

6 ounces fresh snow peas, trimmed

1 can (8¾ ounces) baby corn, rinsed and drained

¼ cup chopped fresh cilantro

2 tablespoons packed brown sugar

2 tablespoons gluten-free fish sauce

1 tablespoon gluten-free soy sauce

1. Heat 3 inches vegetable oil in wok or Dutch oven until oil registers 375°F on deep-fry thermometer. Fry noodles in small batches 20 seconds or until puffy, holding down noodles in oil with slotted spoon or long-handled tongs to fry evenly. Drain on paper towels; set aside.

2. Combine chicken, lemongrass, garlic, ginger, red pepper and black pepper in medium bowl. Blend water and cornstarch in small bowl until smooth; set aside.

3. Heat oil in wok or large skillet over high heat 1 minute. Add chicken mixture; stir-fry 3 minutes or until cooked through.

continued on page 212

gluten-free info

Thin rice noodles are quite versatile. In addition to being soaked and used soft, they can be deep fried for a few seconds until they puff up and become crunchy. The process looks magical. The noodles transform in a matter of seconds, so be prepared to retrieve them with a slotted spoon or tongs and have paper towels ready to drain them.

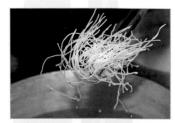
Place noodles in hot oil using long-handled tongs.

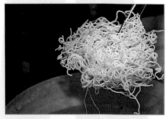
Remove when puffed.

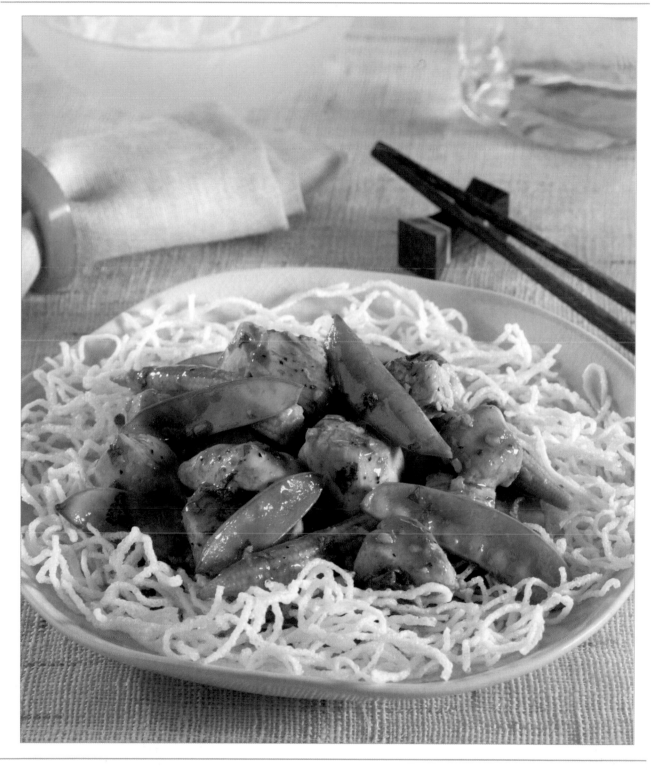

4. Add snow peas and baby corn; stir-fry 1 to 2 minutes. Stir cornstarch mixture; add to wok. Cook 1 minute or until thickened.

5. Add cilantro, brown sugar, fish sauce and soy sauce; cook until heated through. Discard lemongrass. Serve over rice noodles.

Makes 4 servings

midweek moussaka

> **1 eggplant (about 1 pound), cut into ¼-inch slices**
> **2 tablespoons olive oil**
> **1 pound ground beef**
> **1 can (about 14 ounces) stewed tomatoes, drained**
> **¼ cup red wine**
> **2 tablespoons tomato paste**
> **2 teaspoons sugar**
> **¾ teaspoon salt**
> **½ teaspoon dried oregano**
> **¼ teaspoon ground cinnamon**
> **¼ teaspoon black pepper**
> **⅛ teaspoon ground allspice**
> **4 ounces cream cheese**
> **¼ cup milk**
> **¼ cup grated Parmesan cheese**
> **Additional ground cinnamon (optional)**

1. Preheat broiler. Lightly coat 8-inch square baking dish with nonstick cooking spray.

2. Line baking sheet with foil. Arrange eggplant slices on foil, overlapping slightly if necessary. Brush with oil; broil 5 to 6 inches from heat 4 minutes on each side. *Reduce oven temperature to 350°F.*

3. Meanwhile, brown beef in large nonstick skillet over medium-high heat 6 to 8 minutes, stirring to break up meat. Drain fat. Add

recipe notes

Moussaka is a Greek dish made with eggplant and ground lamb or beef. There are many, many variations on the dish made throughout the Mediterranean and Balkan countries. Zucchini or bell peppers can be added and the topping is often custard or white sauce. Moussaka is generally served warm or at room temperature, since it holds together better and is easier to serve once it has cooled slightly.

tomatoes, wine, tomato paste, sugar, salt, oregano, cinnamon, pepper and allspice. Bring to a boil, breaking up large pieces of tomato with spoon. Reduce heat to medium-low; cover and simmer 10 minutes.

4. Place cream cheese and milk in small microwavable bowl. Cover and microwave on HIGH 1 minute.* Stir with fork until smooth.

5. Arrange half of eggplant slices in prepared baking dish. Spoon half of meat sauce over eggplant; sprinkle with half of Parmesan cheese. Repeat layers. Spoon cream cheese mixture evenly over top. Bake 20 minutes or until top begins to crack slightly. Sprinkle lightly with additional cinnamon, if desired. Let stand 10 minutes before serving. *Makes 4 servings*

Or place in small saucepan over medium heat and stir until cream cheese melts.

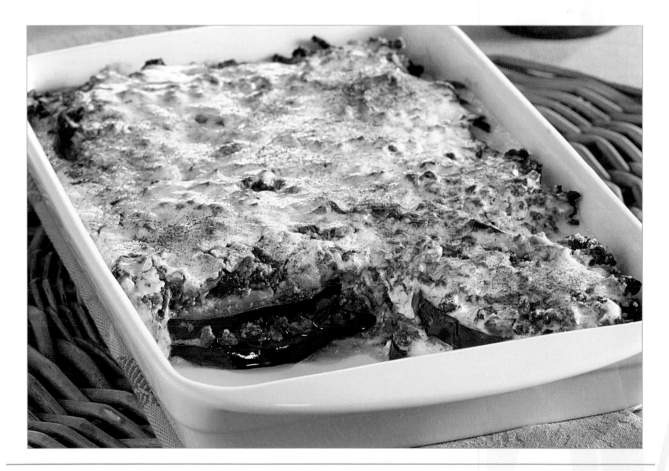

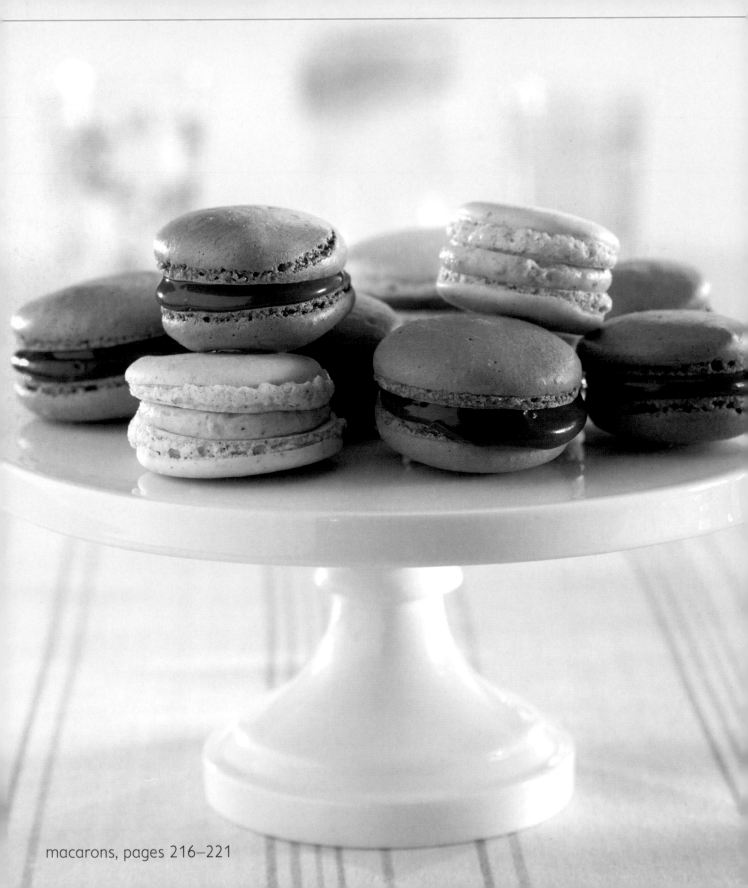

macarons, pages 216–221

sweets & treats

What could be better than homemade cookies? Why gluten-free cookies, of course! Indulge your sweet tooth with desserts of all kinds in every flavor from chocolate to pistachio. Go ahead and try your hand at French macarons. They're beautiful, delicious and naturally gluten-free.

chocolate macarons

1 cup powdered sugar

⅔ cup blanched almond flour (see sidebar)

3 tablespoons unsweetened cocoa powder

3 egg whites, at room temperature*

¼ cup granulated sugar

Chocolate Ganache (page 219), chocolate-hazelnut spread or raspberry jam

For best results, separate the eggs while cold. Leave the egg whites at room temperature for 3 or 4 hours.

1. Line two baking sheets with parchment paper. Double baking sheets by placing another sheet underneath each to prevent macarons from burning or cracking. (Do NOT use insulated baking sheets.)

2. Place powdered sugar, almond flour and cocoa powder in food processor. Pulse 2 to 3 minutes or until well combined into very fine powder, scraping bowl occasionally. *Sift mixture twice.* Discard any remaining large pieces.

3. Beat egg whites in large bowl with electric mixer at high speed until foamy. Gradually add granulated sugar, beating at high speed 2 to 3 minutes until mixture forms stiff, shiny peaks, scraping bowl occasionally.

4. Add half of sifted flour mixture to egg whites. Stir with spatula to combine (about 12 strokes). Repeat with remaining flour mixture. Mix about 15 strokes more by pressing against side of bowl and scooping from bottom until batter is smooth and shiny. Check consistency by dropping spoonful of batter onto plate. It should have a peak which quickly relaxes back into batter. *Do not overmix or undermix.*

5. Attach ½-inch plain piping tip to pastry bag. Scoop batter into bag. Pipe 1-inch circles onto prepared baking sheet about 2 inches apart. Rap baking sheet on flat surface to remove air bubbles and set aside. Repeat with remaining batter. Let macarons rest,

recipe notes

"Macarons" are the French version of macaroons. The more familiar English macaroons are usually made with coconut and egg whites. Macarons and macaroons don't have much in common other than that they are both delicate cookies and naturally gluten-free. Macarons are a bit tricky to make the first time, but fortunately even the ones that don't look perfect still taste delicious. Read through the sidebars accompanying the recipes that follow for tips and hints before beginning.

gluten-free info

Blanched almond flour is available in the specialty flour section of the supermarket or can be ordered on the Internet. Be sure to get very finely ground flour, not coarser almond meal.

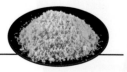

uncovered, until tops harden slightly; this takes from 15 minutes on dry days to 1 hour in more humid conditions. Gently touch top of macaron to check. When batter does not stick, macarons are ready to bake.

6. Meanwhile, preheat oven to 375°F. Place oven rack in center. Place 1 sheet of macarons in oven. *After 5 minutes reduce heat to 325°F.* Bake 10 to 13 minutes, checking at 5 minute intervals. If macarons begin to brown, cover loosely with foil and reduce oven temperature or prop oven open slightly with wooden spoon. Repeat with remaining baking sheet.

7. Cool completely on pan on wire rack. While cooling, if they appear to be sticking to parchment, lift parchment edges and spray pan underneath lightly with water. Steam will help release macarons.

8. Match same size cookies; spread bottom macaron with Chocolate Ganache or raspberry jam and top with another. Store macarons in covered container in refrigerator for 4 to 5 days. Freeze for longer storage.   *Makes 16 to 20 macaron sandwiches*

how-to

Oven temperature is critical for making perfect macarons. Invest in an oven thermometer and check it often while baking. Home ovens are frequently off by 50 degrees. (Yes, even new ovens can be inconsistent.)

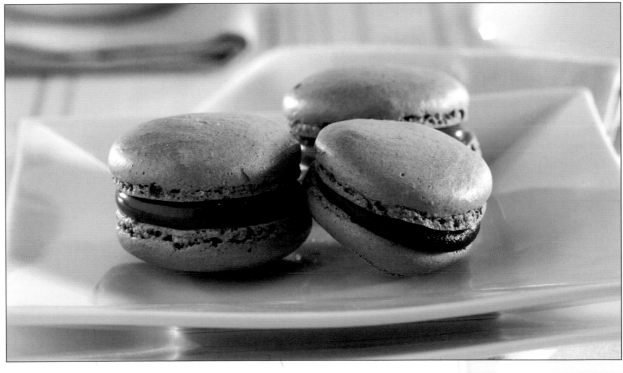

pistachio macarons

⅓ cup unsalted shelled pistachios
1½ cups powdered sugar
⅔ cup blanched almond flour*
3 egg whites, at room temperature**
¼ cup granulated sugar
Green paste food coloring
Chocolate Ganache or Pistachio Filling (page 219)

Almond flour, also called almond powder, is available in the specialty flour section of the supermarket or can be ordered on the Internet.

**For best results, separate the eggs while cold. Leave the egg whites at room temperature for 3 or 4 hours.*

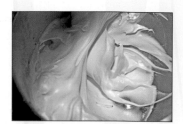
Beat egg whites to stiff peaks.

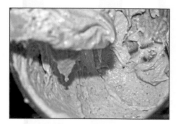
Press batter against sides of bowl until smooth and shiny.

1. Line 2 baking sheets with parchment paper. Double baking sheets by placing another sheet underneath each to prevent macarons from burning or cracking. (Do NOT use insulated baking sheets.)

2. Place pistachios in food processor. Pulse until coarsely ground. Do not overprocess or a paste will form. Add powdered sugar and almond flour. Pulse 2 to 3 minutes or until well combined into very fine powder, scraping bowl occasionally. *Sift mixture twice.* Discard any remaining large pieces.

3. Beat egg whites in large bowl with electric mixer at high speed until foamy. Add food coloring. Gradually add granulated sugar, beating at high speed 2 to 3 minutes until mixture forms stiff, shiny peaks, scraping bowl occasionally.

4. Add half of sifted pistachio mixture to egg whites. Stir with spatula to combine (about 12 strokes). Repeat with remaining pistachio mixture. Mix 15 strokes more by pressing against side of bowl and scooping from bottom, until batter is smooth and shiny. Check consistency by dropping spoonful of batter onto plate. It should have a peak which quickly relaxes back into batter. *Do not overmix or undermix.*

5. Attach ½-inch plain piping tip to pastry bag. Scoop batter into bag. Pipe 1-inch circles onto prepared baking sheet 2 inches apart.

Rap baking sheet on flat surface to remove air bubbles and set aside. Repeat with remaining batter. Let macarons rest, uncovered, until tops harden slightly; this takes from 15 minutes on dry days to 1 hour in more humid conditions. Gently touch top of macaron to check. When batter does not stick, macarons are ready to bake.

6. Meanwhile, preheat oven to 375°F.* Place oven rack in center. Place 1 sheet of macarons in oven. *After 5 minutes reduce heat to 325°F.* Bake 10 to 13 minutes, checking at 5 minute intervals. If macarons begin to brown, cover loosely with foil and reduce oven temperature or prop oven open slightly with wooden spoon. Repeat with remaining baking sheet.

7. Cool completely on pan on wire rack. While cooling, if they appear to be sticking to parchment, lift parchment edges and spray pan underneath lightly with water. Steam will help release macarons.

8. Meanwhile, prepare Pistachio Filling or Chocolate Ganache. When macarons are completely cool, match same size cookies; spread bottom macaron with filling and top with another. Store macarons in covered container in refrigerator for 4 to 5 days. Freeze for longer storage.   *Makes 16 to 20 macaron sandwiches*

Oven temperature is crucial. Use an oven thermometer, if possible.

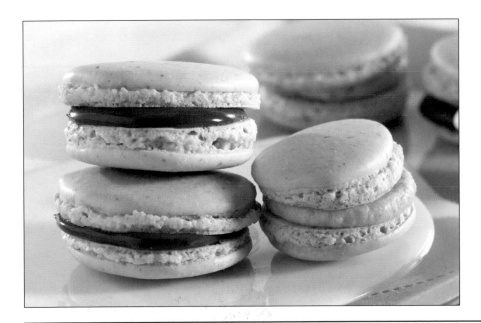

chocolate ganache

Place 4 ounces chopped semisweet or bittersweet chocolate in shallow bowl. Heat ½ cup whipping cream in small saucepan until bubbles form around edges. Pour cream over chocolate; let stand 5 minutes. Stir until smooth.

pistachio filling

Place 1½ ounces pistachios and 1 cup powdered sugar in food processor. Process 2 to 3 minutes or until a coarse paste forms, stopping occasionally to scrape bowl. Add 6 tablespoons softened butter and ½ teaspoon vanilla. Pulse to combine.

raspberry macarons

1½ **cups powdered sugar**

1 **cup blanched almond flour***

3 **egg whites, at room temperature****

¼ **cup granulated sugar**

1 **tablespoon raspberry liqueur**

Red paste food coloring

Raspberry jam or Chocolate Ganache (page 219)

Almond flour, also called almond powder, is available in the specialty flour section of the supermarket or can be ordered on the Internet.

**For best results, separate the eggs while cold. Leave the egg whites at room temperature for 3 or 4 hours. Reserve yolks in refrigerator for another use.*

1. Line two baking sheets with parchment paper. Double baking sheets by placing another sheet underneath each to prevent macarons from burning or cracking. (Do NOT use insulated baking sheets.)

2. Place powdered sugar, almond flour and cocoa powder in food processor. Pulse 2 to 3 minutes or until well combined into very fine powder, scraping bowl occasionally. *Sift mixture twice.* Discard any remaining large pieces.

3. Beat egg whites in large bowl with electric mixer at high speed until foamy. Add liqueur and food coloring. Gradually add granulated sugar, beating at high speed 2 to 3 minutes until mixture forms stiff, shiny peaks, scraping bowl occasionally.

4. Add half of flour mixture to egg whites. Stir with spatula to combine (about 12 strokes). Repeat with remaining flour mixture. Mix 15 strokes more by pressing against side of bowl and scooping from bottom, until batter is smooth and shiny. Check consistency by dropping spoonful of batter onto plate. It should have a peak which quickly relaxes back into batter. *Do not overmix or undermix.*

5. Attach ½-inch plain piping tip to pastry bag. Scoop batter into bag. Pipe 1-inch circles onto prepared baking sheet 2 inches apart. Rap baking sheet on flat surface to remove air bubbles and set

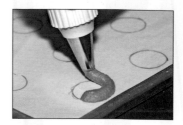

Pipe batter in 1-inch circles. You can make a template as a guide.

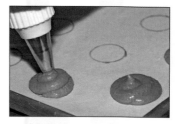

The batter should have a peak when first piped that quickly disappears.

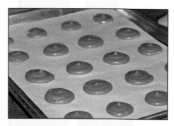

Let macarons rest until tops are dry.

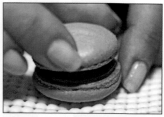

Fill and top with another cookie.

aside. Repeat with remaining batter. Let macarons rest, uncovered, until tops harden slightly; this takes from 15 minutes on dry days to an hour in more humid conditions. Gently touch top of macaron to check. When batter does not stick, macarons are ready to bake.

6. Meanwhile, preheat oven to 375°F.* Place oven rack in center. Place 1 sheet of macarons in oven. *After 5 minutes reduce heat to 325°F.* Bake 10 to 13 minutes, checking at 5 minute intervals. If macarons begin to brown, cover loosely with foil and reduce oven temperature or prop oven open slightly with wooden spoon. Repeat with remaining baking sheet.

7. Cool completely on pan on wire rack. While cooling, if they appear to be sticking to parchment, lift parchment edges and spray pan underneath lightly with water. Steam will help release macarons.

8. Match same size cookies; spread bottom macaron with raspberry jam or Chocolate Ganache and top with another. Store macarons in covered container in refrigerator for 4 to 5 days. Freeze for longer storage.   *Makes 16 to 20 macaron sandwiches*

Oven temperature is crucial. Use an oven thermometer, if possible.

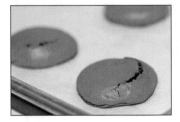

Macarons will crack if oven is too hot or baking sheets are not doubled.

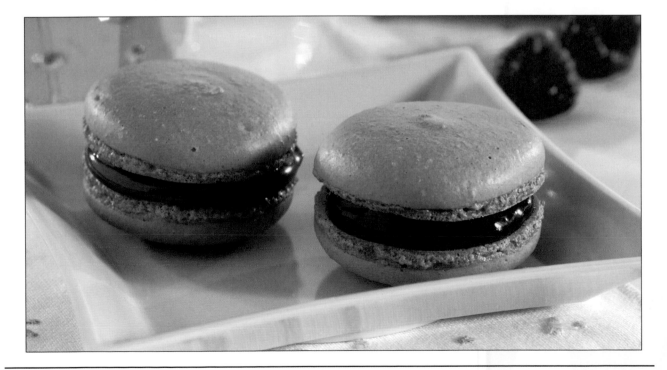

golden kolacky

½ **cup (1 stick) butter, softened**

4 **ounces cream cheese, softened**

1 **cup Gluten-Free All-Purpose Flour Blend (page 19)**

½ **teaspoon xanthan gum**

Fruit preserves

1. Beat butter and cream cheese in large bowl until smooth. Combine flour blend and xanthan gum in medium bowl; gradually add to butter mixture beating until soft dough forms. Divide dough in half; shape into discs. Wrap discs tightly in plastic wrap. Refrigerate about 1 hour or until firm.

2. Preheat oven to 375°F. Roll out dough, one disc at a time, on floured surface to ⅛-inch thickness. Cut into 2½-inch squares. Spoon 1 teaspoon preserves into center of each square. Bring up two opposite corners to center; pinch together tightly to seal. Fold sealed tip to one side. Place 1 inch apart on ungreased cookie sheets.

3. Bake 10 to 15 minutes or until lightly browned. Remove to wire racks; cool completely.   *Makes about 2½ dozen cookies*

recipe notes

Kolacky, also spelled kolache and kolachky, are rich, delicious cookies that are a Polish specialty. Kolacky are traditionally filled with strawberry, apricot, prune, poppy seed or a sweet cheese filling.

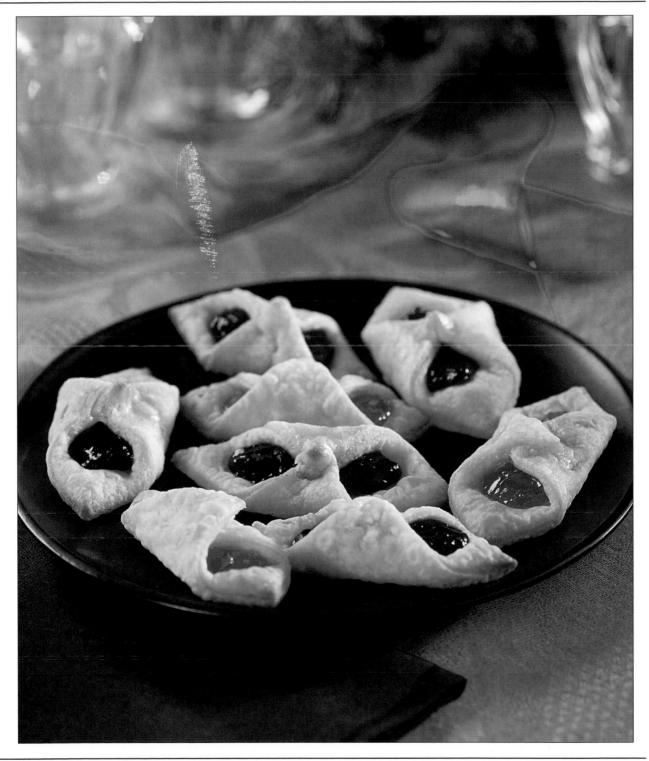

flourless chocolate cake

1 cup whipping cream

1 cup plus 2 tablespoons sugar

12 squares (1 ounce each) unsweetened chocolate, coarsely chopped

4 squares (1 ounce each) semisweet chocolate, coarsely chopped

6 eggs, at room temperature

½ cup strong coffee

¼ teaspoon salt

½ cup chopped walnuts, divided

1. Preheat oven to 350°F; place oven rack in center position. Spray 8-inch round cake pan with nonstick cooking spray.

2. Beat cream with 2 tablespoons sugar in large bowl with electric mixer at high speed until soft peaks form; set aside.

3. Place unsweetened and semisweet chocolate in large microwavable bowl; microwave on HIGH 2 to 3 minutes or until chocolate is melted, stirring after 1 minute and at 30-second intervals after the first minute.

4. Beat eggs and remaining 1 cup sugar in large bowl with electric mixer at high speed about 7 minutes or until pale and thick. Add melted chocolate, coffee and salt; beat until well blended.

5. Fold whipped cream and ¼ cup walnuts into egg mixture. Spread in prepared pan; sprinkle with remaining ¼ cup walnuts. Place pan in large roasting pan; add enough hot water to roasting pan to reach halfway up side of cake pan. Bake 30 to 35 minutes or until set but still soft in center.

6. To unmold, loosen edge of cake with knife; place serving plate upside down over pan and invert. Serve warm.

Makes 12 servings

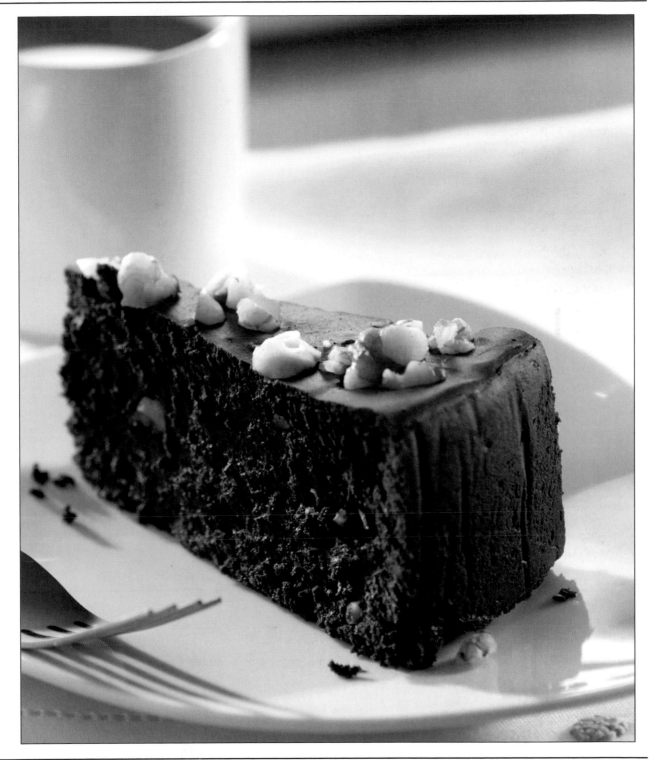

raspberry clafouti

 3 eggs*
 ⅓ cup granulated sugar
 1 cup half-and-half
 2 tablespoons butter, melted and slightly cooled
 ½ teaspoon vanilla
 ⅔ cup almond flour
   Pinch of salt
 2 containers (6 ounces each) fresh raspberries

Use the highest quality eggs possible since the flavor of this dessert depends upon them.

1. Preheat oven to 325°F. Generously butter 9-inch ceramic tart pan or pie plate.

2. Beat eggs and granulated sugar in large bowl with electric mixer at medium speed 3 to 5 minutes or until slightly thickened. Add half-and-half, butter and vanilla; whisk to combine. Gradually whisk in almond flour and salt. Pour enough batter into prepared pan to just cover bottom. Bake 10 minutes or until batter firms.

3. Remove from oven and scatter raspberries over baked batter. Stir remaining batter and pour over raspberries.

4. Return to oven and bake 40 to 45 minutes or until clafouti is set in center and top is golden. Cool on wire rack to room temperature before serving. Refrigerate leftovers.   *Makes 8 to 10 servings*

recipe note

Clafouti is a rustic French dessert that is made by topping fresh fruit with a custard-like batter and baking. The most famous and traditional clafouti is made with cherries, but berries, plums, peaches and pears are also used.

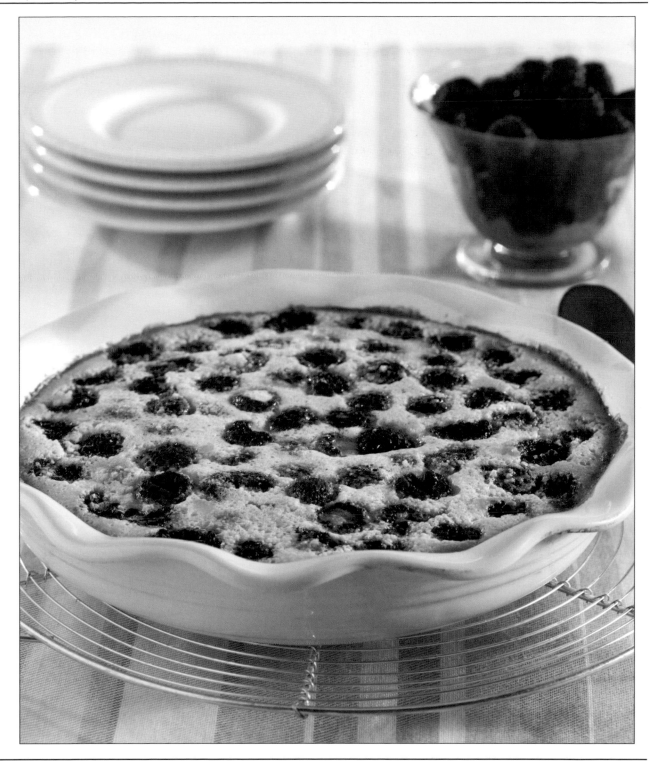

fudge cookies

2 packages (12 ounces each) semisweet chocolate chips, divided

½ cup (1 stick) butter, cut into chunks

2 eggs

1 teaspoon vanilla

¾ cup plus 2 tablespoons sugar

⅔ cup Gluten-Free All-Purpose Flour Blend (page 19)

2 tablespoons unsweetened Dutch process cocoa powder

1 teaspoon baking powder

½ teaspoon xanthan gum

¼ teaspoon salt

1. Line cookie sheets with parchment paper.

2. Combine 1 package chocolate chips and butter in large microwavable bowl. Microwave on HIGH 30 seconds; stir. Repeat as necessary until chips are melted and mixture is smooth. Let cool slightly.

3. Beat eggs and vanilla in large bowl with electric mixer at medium speed until blended and frothy. Add sugar; beat until thick. Add chocolate mixture; beat until well blended. Add flour blend, cocoa, baking powder, xanthan gum and salt; beat until combined. Stir in remaining chocolate chips.

4. Drop dough by rounded tablespoonfuls 1½ inches apart on prepared cookie sheets. Refrigerate 30 minutes.

5. Preheat oven to 325°F. Bake 16 to 20 minutes or until cookies are firm. Cool 2 minutes on cookie sheets. Remove to wire racks; cool completely.   *Makes about 2½ dozen cookies*

dairy-free variation

Replace butter with dairy-free stick margarine (not spread).

gluten-free info

Almost any gluten-free flour or flour blend works well in recipes like this one that only call for a little flour. Do try and convert some of your favorite recipes for regular cookies by substituting a gluten-free flour blend for wheat flour and adding ½ teaspoon of xanthan gum for each cup of flour used. It works especially well for dense cookies that have a lot of flavor from chocolate or spices.

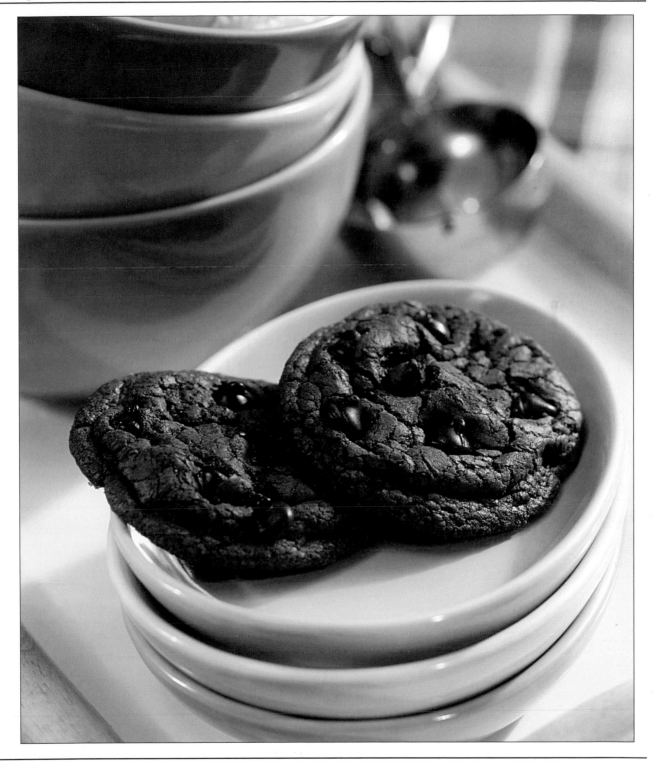

individual orange soufflés

dairy-free

3 oranges
1 tablespoon plus 1½ teaspoons cornstarch
3 tablespoons orange-flavored liqueur
6 egg whites
⅛ teaspoon salt
6 tablespoons granulated sugar
1½ tablespoons sliced almonds (optional)
1½ tablespoons powdered sugar (optional)

1. Preheat oven to 450°F. Spray six individual soufflé dishes, 8 to 10 ounces each, with nonstick cooking spray. Place dishes on jelly-roll pan.

2. Grate enough orange peel to equal 1½ teaspoons. Cut peel and membrane from oranges; section oranges over small saucepan. Dice oranges; add to saucepan. (There will be 1½ cups juice and pulp.) Stir in cornstarch until smooth. Cook and stir over medium heat until mixture comes to a boil and thickens slightly. Remove from heat. Stir in liqueur and orange peel.

3. Beat egg whites and salt in large bowl with electric mixer at high speed until soft peaks form. Beat in granulated sugar, 1 tablespoon at a time, until stiff peaks form. Fold one fourth of egg white mixture into orange mixture. Fold all of orange mixture into remaining egg white mixture. Spoon into prepared dishes. Sprinkle with almonds, if desired.

4. Immediately bake 12 to 15 minutes or until soufflés are puffed and browned. Sprinkle with powdered sugar, if desired. Serve immediately.   *Makes 6 servings*

gluten-free info

Cornstarch is a fine, white powder made from the heart of corn kernels (the endosperm). It is used as a thickener in many recipes and products and also as an ingredient in many gluten-free flour blends. Don't confuse it with cornmeal or corn flour—unless you are in England where cornstarch is called corn flour!

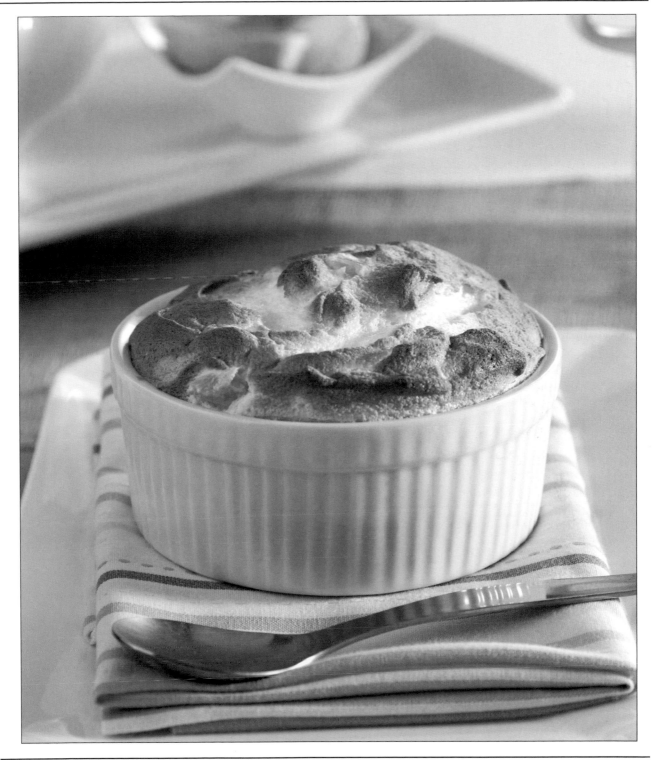

raisin-coconut cookies dairy-free

1¾ cups Gluten-Free All-Purpose Flour Blend (page 19)

2 teaspoons baking powder

½ teaspoon xanthan gum

½ teaspoon salt

1 cup (2 sticks) dairy-free margarine

½ cup granulated sugar

½ cup packed brown sugar

1 egg

1 teaspoon vanilla

2 cups flaked coconut

1½ cups raisins

1. Preheat oven to 350°F. Line cookie sheets with parchment paper.

2. Combine flour blend, baking powder, xanthan gum and salt in medium bowl; whisk to blend.

3. Beat margarine and sugars in large bowl with electric mixer at medium speed about 2 minutes or until well blended. Beat in egg and vanilla. Add flour mixture; beat at low speed about 30 seconds or until just combined. Stir in coconut and raisins. Drop dough by rounded tablespoonfuls 2 inches apart onto prepared cookie sheets.

4. Bake 10 to 12 minutes or until brown around edges (centers will be light). Remove to wire rack; cool completely.

Makes about 4 dozen cookies

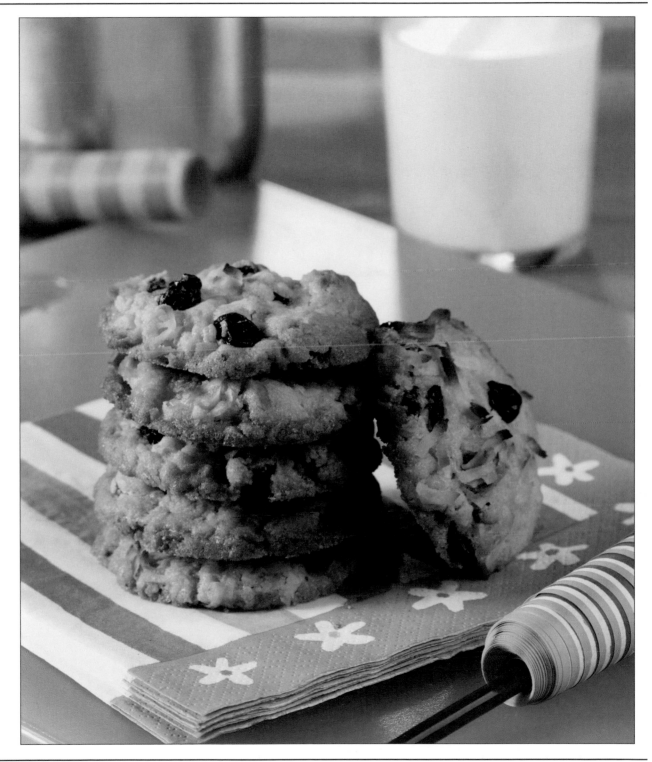

choco-coco pecan crisps

1 cup packed light brown sugar
½ cup (1 stick) butter, softened
1 egg
1 teaspoon vanilla
1½ cups Gluten-Free All-Purpose Flour Blend (page 19)
1 cup chopped pecans
⅓ cup unsweetened cocoa powder
½ teaspoon baking soda
½ teaspoon xanthan gum
1 cup flaked coconut

1. Beat brown sugar and butter in large bowl with electric mixer until light and fluffy. Beat in egg and vanilla. Combine flour blend, pecans, cocoa, baking soda and xanthan gum in small bowl until well blended. Add to butter mixture, blending until stiff dough is formed.

2. Sprinkle coconut on work surface. Divide dough into four pieces. Shape each piece into log about 1½ inches in diameter; roll in coconut until thickly coated. Wrap in plastic wrap; refrigerate until firm, at least 1 hour or up to 2 weeks. (For longer storage, freeze up to 6 weeks.)

3. Preheat oven to 350°F. Cut rolls into ⅛-inch-thick slices. Place 2 inches apart on ungreased cookie sheets. Bake 10 to 13 minutes or until firm. Remove to wire racks; cool completely.

Makes about 6 dozen cookies

dairy-free variation

Replace butter with dairy-free stick margarine (not spread).

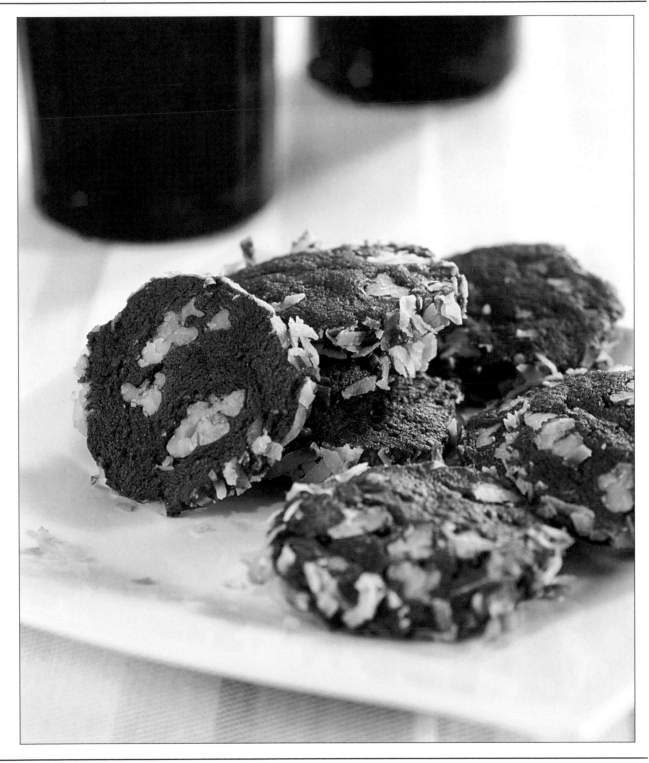

chocolate crème brulée

2 cups whipping cream

3 squares (1 ounce each) semisweet or bittersweet chocolate, finely chopped

3 egg yolks

¼ cup granulated sugar

2 teaspoons vanilla

3 tablespoons brown sugar

1. Preheat oven to 325°F. Heat cream in medium saucepan over medium heat to a simmer (do not boil). Remove from heat; stir in chocolate until melted and smooth. Set aside to cool slightly.

2. Beat egg yolks and granulated sugar in large bowl with electric mixer at medium-high speed about 5 minutes or until mixture is pale and thick. Whisk in chocolate mixture and vanilla until well blended.

3. Divide mixture among four 6-ounce custard cups or individual baking dishes. Place cups in baking pan; place pan in oven. Pour boiling water into baking pan to reach halfway up sides of custard cups. Cover pan loosely with foil.

4. Bake 30 minutes or until edges are just set. Remove cups from baking pan to wire rack; cool completely. Wrap with plastic wrap and refrigerate 4 hours or up to 3 days.

5. When ready to serve, preheat broiler. Spread about 2 teaspoons brown sugar evenly over each cup. Broil 3 to 4 minutes, watching carefully, until sugar bubbles and browns. Serve immediately.

Makes 4 servings

recipe notes

Crème brulée is a dessert many people order in restaurants but don't make at home. That's a pity, because it's actually fairly simple. The only slightly tricky part is browning the sugar on top. You can purchase kitchen torches specially made for crème brulée, or use the broiler. If you use the broiler make sure your dishes can withstand direct heat.

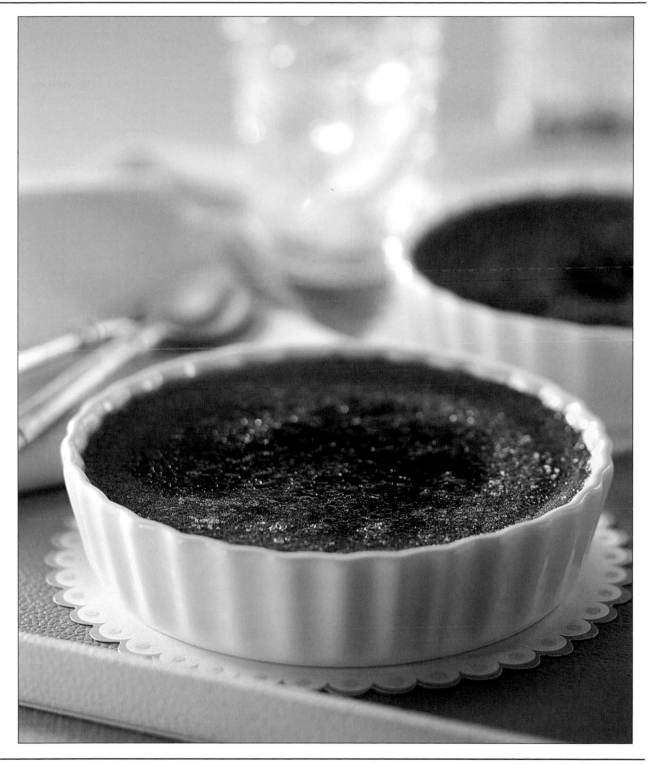

mixed berry crisp

6 cups mixed berries, thawed if frozen
¾ cup packed brown sugar, divided
¼ cup tapioca flour
Juice of ½ lemon
1 teaspoon ground cinnamon
½ cup rice flour
6 tablespoons cold butter, cut into small pieces
½ cup sliced almonds

1. Preheat oven to 375°F. Grease 8- or 9-inch square baking pan.

2. Place berries in large bowl. Add ¼ cup brown sugar, tapioca flour, lemon juice and cinnamon; stir until well combined. Place in prepared pan.

3. Place rice flour, remaining ½ cup brown sugar and butter in food processor. Pulse until mixture resembles coarse crumbs. Add almonds; pulse until combined. (Leave some large pieces of almonds.)

4. Sprinkle almond mixture over berry mixture. Bake 20 to 30 minutes or until golden brown. *Makes 8 servings*

dairy-free variation

Substitute cold dairy-free stick margarine (not spread) for butter.

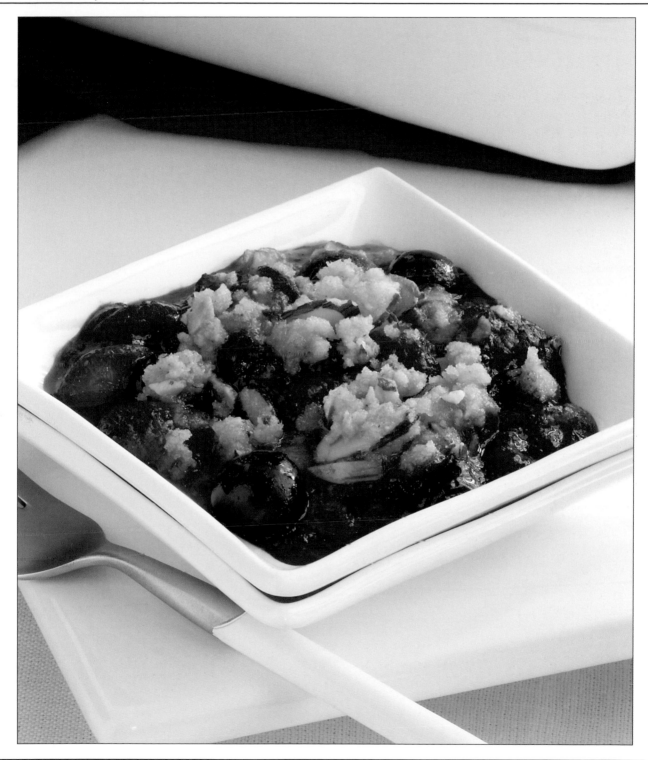

caramel chocolate chunk blondies

dairy-free

1½ cups Gluten-Free All-Purpose Flour Blend (page 19)

1 teaspoon baking powder

½ teaspoon xanthan gum

½ teaspoon salt

¾ cup granulated sugar

¾ cup packed brown sugar

½ cup (1 stick) dairy-free margarine

2 eggs

1½ teaspoons vanilla

1½ cups semisweet chocolate chunks

⅓ cup caramel ice cream topping

1. Preheat oven to 350°F. Spray 13×9-inch baking pan with nonstick cooking spray.

2. Combine flour blend, baking powder, xanthan gum and salt in medium bowl. Beat granulated sugar, brown sugar and margarine in large bowl with electric mixer at medium speed until smooth and creamy. Beat in eggs and vanilla until well blended. Add flour mixture; beat at low speed until blended. Stir in chocolate chunks.

3. Spread batter evenly in prepared pan. Drop spoonfuls of caramel topping over batter; swirl into batter with knife.

4. Bake 25 minutes or until golden brown. Cool completely in pan on wire rack.   *Makes about 2½ dozen blondies*

caramel chocolate chunk blondies

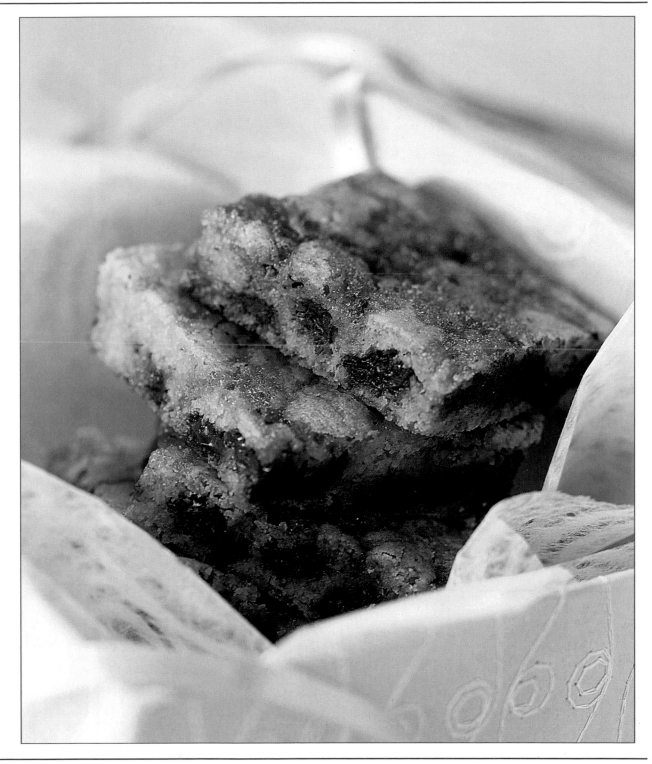

cranberry-orange rice pudding

1 cup uncooked rice*
1 tablespoon grated orange peel
1½ cups dried cranberries, coarsely chopped
½ cup orange juice
1 quart (4 cups) milk
1 can (12 ounces) evaporated milk
⅔ cup sugar
⅛ teaspoon salt

*Or substitute 1½ cups converted rice or 3 cups cooked rice.

1. Cook rice according to package directions adding orange peel.

2. Meanwhile, combine cranberries and orange juice in medium saucepan; bring to a simmer over medium heat. Simmer until juice is absorbed. Set aside.

3. Add milk, evaporated milk, sugar and salt to cooked rice. Cook and stir over medium-low heat about 40 minutes or until slightly thickened.

4. Stir cranberries into rice mixture. Cool to room temperature. Cover; refrigerate. Let stand at room temperature 10 minutes before serving. *Makes 8 servings*

gluten-free info

The many varieties of rice are usually classified by the size of the grain—short, medium or long. Long-grain rice cooks up fluffy and dry, so it is good as a side dish or to serve under a saucy main course. Varieties of long-grain rice include fragrant basmati and jasmine. Medium-grain rice is shorter and clumps together a bit more when cooked. Short-grain rice has plump grains that can be almost round. They release more starch during cooking and so the grains stick together. Most Asian varieties, like those for sushi, are short grain. Rice that clumps is easier to eat with chopsticks. Any variety may be used for rice pudding, but short-grain will produce a creamier dessert.

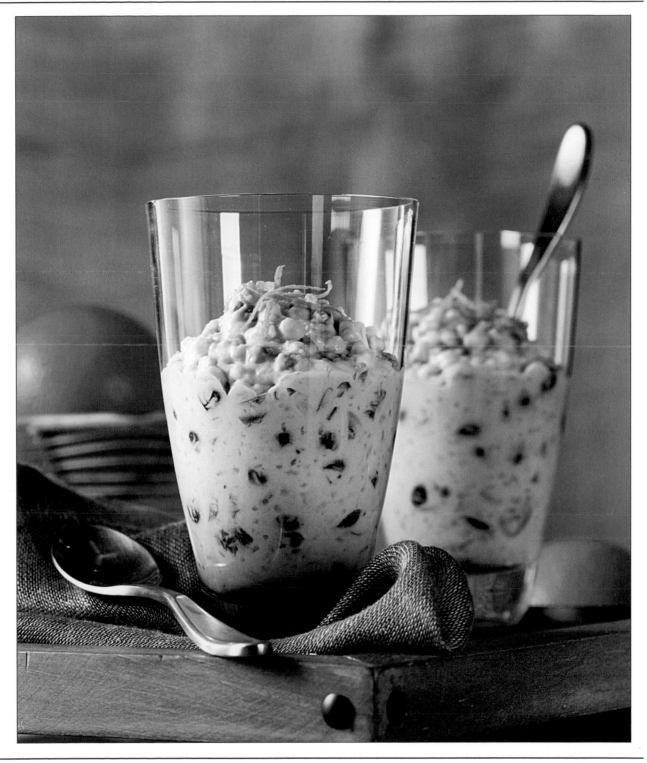

flourless peanut butter cookies dairy-free

1 cup packed light brown sugar
1 cup smooth peanut butter
1 egg, lightly beaten
½ cup dairy-free semisweet chocolate chips, melted

1. Preheat oven to 350°F. Beat brown sugar, peanut butter and egg in medium bowl with electric mixer until blended and smooth.

2. Shape dough into 24 (1½-inch) balls; place 2 inches apart on ungreased cookie sheets. Flatten dough slightly with fork. Bake 10 to 12 minutes or until set. Remove to wire racks; cool completely. Drizzle with chocolate.   *Makes 2 dozen cookies*

flourless almond cookies

dairy-free

1 cup sugar
1 cup almond butter
1 egg, lightly beaten

1. Preheat oven to 350°F. Beat sugar, almond butter and egg in large bowl with electric mixer until blended and smooth.

2. Shape dough into 24 balls; place 2 inches apart on ungreased cookie sheets. Flatten slightly with fork.

3. Bake 10 minutes or until set. Remove to wire rack; cool completely.   *Makes 2 dozen cookies*

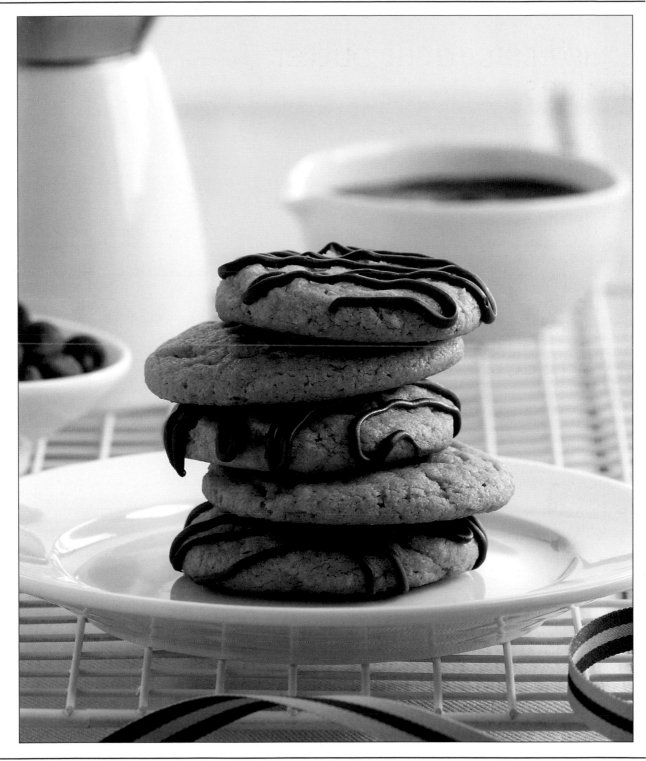

cocoa raisin-chip cookies

 dairy-free

1½ cups **Gluten-Free All-Purpose Flour Blend (page 19)**

¼ cup **unsweetened cocoa powder**

1 teaspoon **baking powder**

½ teaspoon **salt**

¼ teaspoon **xanthan gum**

1 cup **packed light brown sugar**

½ cup **granulated sugar**

½ cup (1 stick) **dairy-free margarine**

½ cup **shortening**

2 **eggs**

1 teaspoon **vanilla**

1½ cups **dairy-free semisweet chocolate chips**

1 cup **raisins**

¾ cup **chopped walnuts**

1. Preheat oven to 350°F. Line cookie sheets with parchment paper.

2. Combine flour blend, cocoa, baking powder, salt and xanthan gum in medium bowl. Beat brown sugar, granulated sugar, margarine and shortening in large bowl with electric mixer at medium speed until light and creamy. Add eggs, one at a time, beating well after each addition. Beat in vanilla. Add flour mixture; beat until well blended. Stir in chocolate chips, raisins and walnuts. Drop dough by tablespoonfuls onto prepared cookie sheets.

3. Bake 10 to 12 minutes or until set. Remove to wire racks; cool completely. *Makes about 4 dozen cookies*

allergy info

Chocolate chips are gluten-free, but many varieties are not dairy-free, so check labels carefully if this is a dietary concern. Obviously milk chocolate chips contain dairy, but some semisweet chips also contain casein or other dairy ingredients.

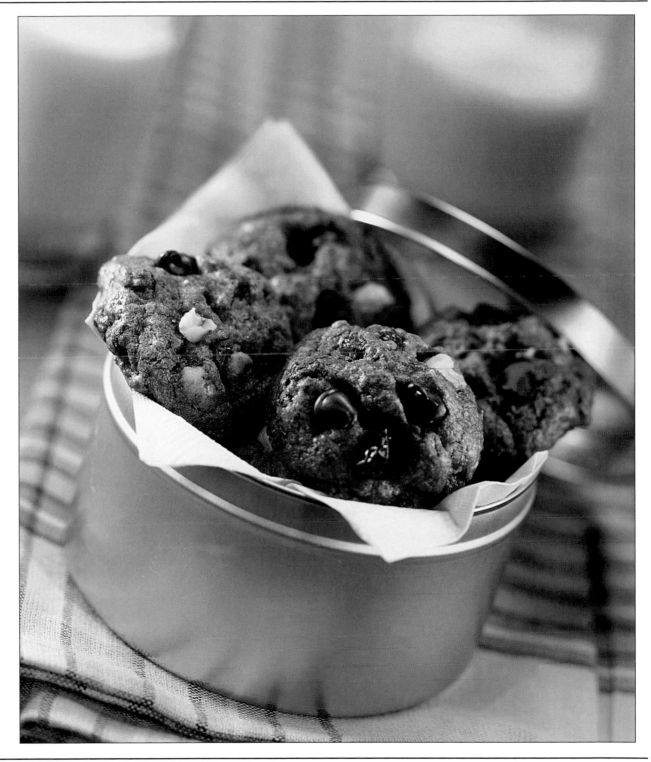

cocoa bottom banana pecan bars

 dairy-free

 1 cup sugar
 ½ cup (1 stick) dairy-free margarine
 5 ripe bananas, mashed
 1 egg
 1 teaspoon vanilla
 1½ cups Gluten-Free All-Purpose Flour Blend (page 19)
 1 teaspoon baking powder
 1 teaspoon baking soda
 ½ teaspoon xanthan gum
 ½ teaspoon salt
 ½ cup chopped pecans
 ¼ cup unsweetened cocoa powder

1. Preheat oven to 350°F. Grease 13×9-inch baking pan.

2. Beat sugar and margarine in large bowl with electric mixer at medium speed until creamy. Add bananas, egg and vanilla; beat until well blended. Combine flour blend, baking powder, baking soda, xanthan gum and salt in medium bowl. Add to banana mixture; beat until well blended. Stir in pecans.

3. Remove half of batter to another bowl; stir in cocoa. Spread chocolate batter in prepared pan. Top with plain batter; swirl with knife.

4. Bake 30 to 35 minutes or until edges are lightly browned. Cool completely in pan on wire rack. Cut into bars.

Makes 2 dozen bars

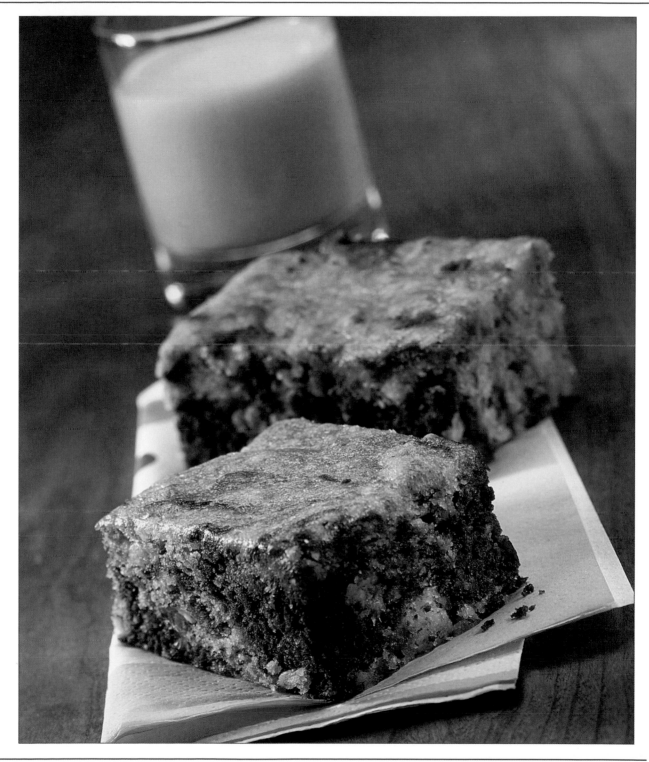

index

metric
conversion chart

VOLUME MEASUREMENTS (dry)

⅛ teaspoon = 0.5 mL
¼ teaspoon = 1 mL
½ teaspoon = 2 mL
¾ teaspoon = 4 mL
1 teaspoon = 5 mL
1 tablespoon = 15 mL
2 tablespoons = 30 mL
¼ cup = 60 mL
⅓ cup = 75 mL
½ cup = 125 mL
⅔ cup = 150 mL
¾ cup = 175 mL
1 cup = 250 mL
2 cups = 1 pint = 500 mL
3 cups = 750 mL
4 cups = 1 quart = 1 L

VOLUME MEASUREMENTS (fluid)

1 fluid ounce (2 tablespoons) = 30 mL
4 fluid ounces (½ cup) = 125 mL
8 fluid ounces (1 cup) = 250 mL
12 fluid ounces (1½ cups) = 375 mL
16 fluid ounces (2 cups) = 500 mL

WEIGHTS (mass)

½ ounce = 15 g
1 ounce = 30 g
3 ounces = 90 g
4 ounces = 120 g
8 ounces = 225 g
10 ounces = 285 g
12 ounces = 360 g
16 ounces = 1 pound = 450 g

DIMENSIONS

1/16 inch = 2 mm
⅛ inch = 3 mm
¼ inch = 6 mm
½ inch = 1.5 cm
¾ inch = 2 cm
1 inch = 2.5 cm

OVEN TEMPERATURES

250°F = 120°C
275°F = 140°C
300°F = 150°C
325°F = 160°C
350°F = 180°C
375°F = 190°C
400°F = 200°C
425°F = 220°C
450°F = 230°C

BAKING PAN SIZES

Utensil	Size in Inches/Quarts	Metric Volume	Size in Centimeters
Baking or Cake Pan (square or rectangular)	8×8×2	2 L	20×20×5
	9×9×2	2.5 L	23×23×5
	12×8×2	3 L	30×20×5
	13×9×2	3.5 L	33×23×5
Loaf Pan	8×4×3	1.5 L	20×10×7
	9×5×3	2 L	23×13×7
Round Layer Cake Pan	8×1½	1.2 L	20×4
	9×1½	1.5 L	23×4
Pie Plate	8×1¼	750 mL	20×3
	9×1¼	1 L	23×3
Baking Dish or Casserole	1 quart	1 L	—
	1½ quart	1.5 L	—
	2 quart	2 L	—